RETINITIS PIGMENTOSA: CAUSES, DIAGNOSIS AND TREATMENT

EYE AND VISION RESEARCH DEVELOPMENTS SERIES

Eye Cancer Research Progress
Edwin B. Bospene (Editor)
2008. ISBN: 978-1-60456-045-9

Non-Age Related Macular Degeneration
Enzo B. Mercier
2008. ISBN: 978-1-60456-305-4

Optic Nerve Disease Research Perspectives
Benjamin D. Lewis and Charlie James Davies (Editors)
2008. ISBN: 978-1-60456-490-7

Optic Nerve Disease Research Perspectives
Benjamin D. Lewis and Charlie James Davies (Editors)
2008. ISBN: 978-1-60741-938-9 (Online book)

New Topics in Eye Research
Lauri Korhonen and Elias Laine (Editors)
2009. ISBN: 978-1-60456-510-2

Eye Infections, Blindness and Myopia
Jeffrey Higgins and Dominique Truax (Editors)
2009. ISBN: 978-1-60692-630-7

Eye Research Developments:
Glaucoma, Corneal Transplantation, and Bacterial Eye Infections
Alan N. Westerhouse (Editor)
2009. ISBN: 978-1-60741-1772

Retinal Degeneration: Causes, Diagnosis and Treatment
Robert B. Catlin (Editor)
2009. ISBN: 978-1-60741-007-2

Retinal Degeneration: Causes, Diagnosis and Treatment
Robert B. Catlin (Editor)
2009. ISBN: 978-1-60876-442-6 (Online book)

Binocular Vision: Development, Depth Perception and Disorders
Jacques McCoun and Lucien Reeves (Editors)
2010. ISBN: 978-1-60876-547-8

**Understanding Corneal Biomechanics through Experimental
Assessment and Numerical Simulation**
Ahmed Elsheikh
2010. ISBN: 978-1-60876-694-9

Retinitis Pigmentosa: Causes, Diagnosis and Treatment
Michaël Baert and Cédric Peeters (Editors)
2010. ISBN: 978-1-60876-884-4

Color: Ontological Status and Epistemic Role
Anna Storozhuk
2010. ISBN: 978-1-61668-201-9

Color: Ontological Status and Epistemic Role
Anna Storozhuk
2010. ISBN: 978-1-61668-608-6 (Online book)

Coherent Effects in Primary Visual Perception
V.D. Svet and A.M. Khazen
2010. ISBN: 978-1-61668-143-2

Coherent Effects in Primary Visual Perception
V.D. Svet and A.M. Khazen
2010. ISBN: ISBN: 978-1-61668-496-9 (Online book)

Conjunctivitis: Symptoms, Treatment and Prevention
Anna R. Sallinger
2010. ISBN: 978-1-61668-321-4

Conjunctivitis: Symptoms, Treatment and Prevention
Anna R. Sallinger
2010. ISBN: 978-1-61668-443-3 (Online book)

EYE AND VISION RESEARCH DEVELOPMENTS SERIES

RETINITIS PIGMENTOSA: CAUSES, DIAGNOSIS AND TREATMENT

MICHAËL BAERT
AND
CÉDRIC PEETERS
EDITORS

Nova Biomedical Books
New York

NOTICE TO THE READER

Library of Congress Cataloging-in-Publication Data

Retinitis pigmentosa : causes, diagnosis, and treatment / editors, Michaël Baert and Cédric Peeters.
    p. ; cm.
 Includes bibliographical references and index.
 ISBN 978-1-60876-884-4 (softcover : alk. paper)
 1. Retinitis pigmentosa. I. Baert, Michaël. II. Peeters, Cédric.
 [DNLM: 1. Retinitis Pigmentosa--etiology. 2. Retinitis Pigmentosa--diagnosis.
3. Retinitis Pigmentosa--therapy. WW 270 R438895 2009]
 RE661.R45R467 2009
 617.7'35--dc22
                          2009045932

Published by Nova Science Publishers, Inc. ✦ New York

Contents

Preface

Retinis Pigmentosa (RP) includes a group of progressive hereditary retinal diseases involving degeneration of rod and cone photoreceptors, predominantly the former, and is one of the leading causes of hereditary blindness in the developed world. Clinical symptoms include nyctalopia, progressive visual field loss, and deterioration in visual acuity in adolescence. It affects one in 3000-5000 individuals and can be caused by mutations in more than 40 genes. In addition, Retinitis Pigmentosa may exist either alone (nonsyndromic) or as part of a neurological or systemic disorder, such as Usher's syndrome and Infantile Refsum's disease. There are few effective clinical treatments for retinitis pigmentosa which affects an estimated 1.5 million individuals worldwide. However, understanding the histopathologic changes occurring in RP is critical to understanding the rationale for current therapies, as well as to develop future therapies. This book highlights the most recent research done in the field.

Chapter I - Retinitis Pigmentosa is one of the leading causes of blindness worldwide and lacks effective clinical treatment. Stem cell-based therapy offers a novel experimental therapeutic approach, based on the strategy that transplanted progenitor cells could replace damaged photoreceptor cells. However, it is still unknown what is the optimal time to choose for targeting the host tissue during the progression of the degeneration, the characteristics and potential capacities in different stem cells, whether stem cells differentiate into functional daughter cells, and the degree to which host retinal function can be restored.

We have used Royal College of Surgeons (RCS) rats as a suitable model of retinitis pigmentosa and light induced photorecptor damage in minipigs to study the effectiveness of cell transplant therapies and the functional capcity of the retina. Initially, whole-cell patch clamp studies showed three action potential discharge patterns of retinal ganglion cells (RGCs) in RCS rats: single, transient, and sustained firing. The main discharge pattern was single firing between postnatal weeks 1 and 2 (P1-2W), followed later by transient and sustained firing patterns. However, during later stages of retinal degeneration at P7-8W, 26.7% RGCs lack action potentials in RCS rats, and this proportion had increased (63.2% of RGCs) by P9-12W. This suggested functional RGCs were maintained in the early stages of retinal degeneration, but this functional parameter was lost during retinal degeneration, even though morphological differences are not apparent. Cultured stem cells from embryonic rat retina differentiated and produced action potentials in vitro showing that the maturation of electrophysiological properties of presumptive RGCs occurs after at least 15 days under culture conditions. Knowledge of the timing of voltage-dependent ion channel development provides a time window stem cell funcitonal matureation that will help to improve success rate in transplantation protocols if functional recouvery is to be achieved. We found that, three types of stem cells (rat optic cup at embryonic day 12.5 (OC-RSCs), retinal stem cells from embryonic day 17 induced by BDNF (RSCs–BDNF) and rat bone marrow stromal cells (BMSCs)) were incorporated into the degenerating retina and differentiated into rhodopsin positive cells. Thus, all three stem cell types are suitable for retinal transplantation, although RSCs from different developmental stages have distinct proliferative capacities and differentiation potential. OC-RSCs are easier to passage, although a large number of E12.5 embryos are required. BMSCs are easier to obtain and can restore retinal function in RCS rats for up to two months after transplantation. The retinal transplantation in minipigs by neonatal pig retina or human fetal retina with an intact retinal pigment epithelium (RPE) was successful in 66.7% of the experiments. Twelve months follow up showed that xenografts transplantation had not resulted in any immunological rejection and thus was a safe technique. After the human fetal retina transplantation, the grafts survived and retained characteristics of progenitor precursor cells, such as Chx10 labeling. Multifocal electroretinography (mfERG) showed improvement of central posterior retinal function from the 1st to 8th month after transplantation. Müller cells are an integral and important glial component in the normal function of the retina and form an vital part of the regenertive process. Immunocytochemistry showed that Müller cells express retinal progenitor cell markers during chronic retina degeneration. After RSC transplantation, Müller cells were seen to differentiate into photoreceptors within and nearby the grafted area. This suggests that Müller cells have the potential to re-enter the cell cycle and can differentiate into host photoreceptor cells thus restoring lost retinal components. Further studies are needed to determine how to maintain the progenitor potential of Müller cells and how RCS transplants may augment this process of restoring cells, especially photoreceptors, to the damaged retina. These studies may help to understand how host retinal function can be restored with these combined techniques.

Chapter II - Retinis Pigmentosa (RP) is a term that includes a group of progressive hereditary retinal diseases involving degeneration of rod and cone photoreceptors, predominantly the former, and is one of the leading causes of hereditary blindness in the developed world. Ganglion cells are also affected, possibly due to transsynaptic neuronal damage caused by loss of neuronal input from the degenerating photoreceptor cell layer. Clinical symptoms include nyctalopia, progressive visual field loss, and deterioration in visual acuity in adolescence. No effective therapy exists at present. It affects one in 3000-5000 individuals and can be caused by mutations in more than 40 genes. Retinitis Pigmentosa may exist either alone (nonsyndromic) or as part of a neurological or systemic disorder, such as Usher's syndrome and Infantile Refsum's disease. Typical findings on retinal examination include retinal vessel attenuation. Bone spicule formation is also noted around the intraretinal vessels (pigmentary clumping), caused by the hyperplasia and migration of retinal pigment epithelial cells into the inner layers of the neurosensory retina. The disease may be inherited as either autosomal recessive, autosomal dominant or X-linked. Autosomal dominant inheritance is the most common. Several mechanisms to explain the degeneration process have been proposed. These include misfolding of the rod visual pigment Rhodopsin preventing its transportation to the outer segment, dysfunction of cell transport systems that are involved with photoreceptor protein localization, starvation of cones and cyclic GMP-dependent protein kinase activation. Therapies that are currently under investigation include the use of ribozymes for the targeted reduction of mutant-allele mRNA and the use of retinoids to improve protein folding.

Chapter III - Recently, *RPE65* gene replacement therapy in a total of nine human subjects with Leber congenital amaurosis marked the first treatment for genetic retinal degenerative diseases (RDD). The prospect of imminent gene therapy made *RPE65* a strong candidate for mutation screening in South Africa. An added impetus for this study was the fact that a founder mutation in *RPE65* was described as causing an early onset RDD in an isolated Dutch population, and the founder effect in South Africans descended from Dutch settlers has been well documented for other diseases and genes.

Mutations in the *RPE65* gene are reported to be responsible for approximately 2% of autosomal recessive retinitis pigmentosa (arRP) and 16% of Leber congenital amaurosis (LCA). For this study a cohort of 87 affected, unrelated individuals was selected for mutation screening. Of these individuals, 18 were classified as having LCA and 69 as having early onset RP (with an age of onset younger than 15 years). Of the LCA cohort, 4 exhibited autosomal recessive inheritance (arLCA) and 14 were isolated cases. Of the RP cohort, 44 had arRP and 25 were isolated cases. The ethnic breakdown of the cohort was as follows: 65 were Caucasian, 7 were indigenous Black African, 10 of Asian Indian origin, 4 of Mixed Ancestry (comprising individuals whose ancestry is a mixture of Caucasian, Malaysian, Madagascan and indigenous African including Khoi-San and West African) and 1 was Taiwanese. The 14 exons of *RPE65*, including the intron/exon boundaries, were screened using denaturing high performance liquid chromatography (dHPLC) analysis and variations were characterised by direct sequencing.

Five different pathogenic mutations (of which 2 were novel) were identified in the cohort of 69 individuals diagnosed with early onset RP. The Dutch founder mutation, Tyr368His, was the only homozygous mutation detected and was identified in a family of Mixed Ancestry with arRP. In two families, compound heterozygous mutations in *RPE65* are presumed to be causative of disease: Ala132Thr and the novel IVS1+1G>T mutation was present in one Indian family with arRP; Leu22Pro and the novel Glu21Lys mutation were present in one Caucasian individual with isolated RP. In two cases (one Indian family with arRP and one Caucasian individual with isolated RP) a single heterozygous Ala132Thr mutation was identified and the second mutation, should it exist, is unknown. This Ala132Thr mutation was the single most common variation detected, as it was identified in three of the 69 individuals classified as having RP (4.4%). No pathogenic mutations were identified in the cohort of patients diagnosed with LCA.

The identification of disease-causing genetic mutations in families with RDD generally means that predictive, diagnostic and prenatal testing can be offered to family members, although few options exist for treatment. Importantly, three families in South Africa possibly stand to benefit from therapeutic intervention by *RPE65* gene replacement therapy.

Chapter IV - Retinitis pigmentosa (RP) is a group of inherited retinal degenerations, caused by mutations in one of many genes - some already identified, and some still yet to be discovered. While there are many different genes involved and great heterogeneity among these genes, the underlying common source of vision loss is retinal dysfunction related to photoreceptor loss. The sequence of histopathologic changes associated with RP occurs in several stages. The 1st stage is associated with rod photoreceptor dysfunction and ultimate death and the second with cone photoreceptor demise. Following photoreceptor loss, a number of secondary changes occur, with retinal pigment epithelial (RPE) cells detaching from of Bruch's membrane and migrating into the inner retina to ultimately accumulate and surround blood vessels which gives rise to the "bone spicules" observed clinically. Other pathologies include attenuation of blood vessels, retinal gliosis, migration of microglia into the outer retina, optic nerve atrophy and mild vitritis. Current therapies for RP include: genetic replacement of missing/mutated proteins via viral vectors, addition (by injection or surgery) of factors or supplements that may prolong photoreceptor survival, transplantation of photoreceptors and RPE cells and electrical stimulation of remaining neurons, as well as developing therapies targeted at preventing photoreceptor apoptosis. Understanding the histopathologic changes occurring in RP is critical to understanding the rationale for current therapies, as well as to develop future therapies. Mouse models of retinitis pigmentosa, have been instrumental in aiding the study of histopathologic changes that occur in the setting of retinitis pigmentosa and to initiate and study various treatment approaches. Many of the findings of the histopathologic changes and treatment avenues are explored in these models.

Chapter V - We identified mutations in the RHO and RDS genes in patients with autosomal dominant and sporadic forms of retinitis pigmentosa (RP) from Volga-Ural region of Russia. The 5 exons of RHO and 3 exons of RDS genes were analyzed for sequence changes by single-strand conformation polymorphism (SSCP) and direct sequencing. Patients were examined clinically and with visual function tests. We detected known mutation Pro347Leu and novel mutation Arg252Pro and two polymorphisms IVS1+10g>a, IVS3+4c>t in RHO gene. There were statistically significant differences in allele and genotype frequencies of sequence change IVS3+4c>t of RHO gene in affected patients with RP and in controls. According to our data, this polymorphism is likely to be pathogenic. Recently were reported 16 possible combinations of the exon 3 RDS gene SNPs and detected four from 16 possible combinations (minihaplotypes): $G^{1147}A^{1166}G^{1250}C^{1291}$ (I),

$C^{1147}A^{1166}A^{1250}C^{1291}$ (II), $C^{1147}G^{1166}A^{1250}C^{1291}$ (III) and $G^{1147}A^{1166}G^{1250}T^{1291}$ (IV). Telmer C.A. 2003 established that minihaplotype $C^{1147}A^{1166}A^{1250}C^{1291}$ (II) was linked to the mutation IVS2+3a>t. Sequencing results for variant positions in exon 3 RDS gene in RP patients from Volga-Ural region showed all four minihaplotypes described above and minihaplotype $C^{1147}A^{1166}A^{1250}T^{1291}$ (V). Our study determined that minihaplotype $C^{1147}A^{1166}A^{1250}C^{1291}$ (II) isn't linked to mutation IVS2+3a>t in adRP and sporadic RP patients from Volga-Ural region. To optimize the DNA diagnostics of retinitis pigmentosa, it is necessary to analyze patients from various ethnic groups. Our study helps in molecular characterization of RP in Russia.

Chapter VI - The rd1 (retinal degeneration) mouse retina shows degeneration homologous to a form of retinitis pigmentosa with a rapid loss of rod photoreceptors and deficiency of retinal blood vessels. Due to Pde6brd1 gene mutation, β subunit of phosphodiesterase (PDE) of rd1 retina has an inactive PDE which elevates cGMP and Ca2+ ions level. In vitro retinal explants provide a system close to the in vivo situation, so both approaches were used to compare the status of oxidative stress, transforming growth factor-β1

(TGF-β1), sialylation, galactosylation of proteoglycans, and different proteinases-endogenous inhibitors systems participating in extracellular matrix (ECM) remodeling/degeneration and programmed cell death (PCD)/apoptosis in wt and rd1 mouse retinas.

Proteins and desialylated sulfated glucosaminoglycan parts of proteoglycans in ECM of rd1 retina were, respectively, decreased and increased due to enhanced activities of proteinases. Desialylation increases the susceptibility of cells to phoagocytosis/ apoptosis, decreased neurogenesis and faulty guidance cues for synaptogenesis. In vivo activities of total proteinases, matrix metalloproteinase-9 (MMP-9) and cathepsin B were increased in rd1 retina on postnatal day 14 (PN14), -21 and -28, due to relatively lower levels of tissue inhibitor of MMPs (TIMP-1) and cystatin C, respectively. This corresponded with increased in vitro secretion of these proteinases by rd1 retina. Cells including end-feet of Mueller cells in degenerating rd1 retina showed intense immunolabeling for MMP-9, MMP-2/TIMP-1, TIMP-2 and cathepsin B/cystatin C, and proteinases pool was increased by Mueller cells. Intense immunolabeling of ganglion cell (RGC) layer for cathepsin B and of inner-plexiform layer of both PN2/PN7 rd1 and wt retinas indicated importance of cathepsin B in synaptogenesis and PCD of RGC.

Increased levels of TGF-β1 **in vitro** transiently increased the secretion of MMPs and cathepsins activities by wt explants which activate TGF-β1 **and** remodel the ECM for angiogenesis and ontogenetic PCD. Whereas, lower level of TGF-β1 **and persistently higher activities of MMPs and** cathepsins in rd1 retinas and conditioned medium, suggested that proteinases degraded TGF-β1 **and ECM and caused retinal degeneration.**

Lower activities of glutathione-S-transferase and glutathione-peroxidase in rd1 retina contribute to oxidative stress which damages membranes and increased the expression, release/secretion of proteinases relative to their endogenous inhibitors. Participation of oxidative stress in rd1 retinal degeneration was further confirmed from the partial protection of rd1 photoreceptors by in vitro and/or in vivo supplementation with glutathione-S-transferase or a combination of antioxidants namely lutein, **zeaxanthin,** α-lipoic acid and reduced-L-glutathione. Treatment with combination(s) of broad spectrum proteinase inhibitor(s) and antioxidants needs investigation.

Chapter VII - The aim of our study was to ascertain if visual training by means of Visual Pathfinder (LACE inc.) biofeedback system could be successful to improve and/or restore visual function in visually impaired patients with retinitis pigmentosa.

We enrolled 15 patients (age range 8-55) and examined a total of 30 eyes with retinitis pigmentosa. All the patients underwent a complete ophthalmologic evaluation which comprised the assessment of best corrected visual acuity (BCVA) and pattern reversal visual evoked potential (VEP) according to the ISCEV standards. All the patients underwent 10 training sessions of 10 minutes each eye performed once a week using the Visual Pathfinder.

Statistical analysis was performed using the Student's t-test. P values less than 0.05 were considered statistically significant.

The mean BCVA was 0.67 ± 0.14 logMAR at the baseline assessment, and 0.84 ± 0.11 logMAR at the end of visual training; this result was statistically significant (p=0.035). VEP amplitude of P100 wave was 2.14 ± 0.88 mV at the baseline assessment, and 4.86 ± 1.12 mV at the end of visual training; this result was statistically significant (p=0.012).

In conclusion our experience demonstrates that visual training by means of a visual evoked acoustic biofeedback with Visual Pathfinder can significantly improve visual acuity and pattern reversal VEP amplitude in retinitis pigmentosa, resulting in more suitable visual performances, better

quality of life, and a much more positive psychological situation for these
patients.

In: Reginitis Pigmentosa: Causes, Diagnosis...   ISBN: 978-1-60876-884-4
Editors: M. Baert, et al. pp. 1-63   © 2010 Nova Science Publishers, Inc.

Chapter I

Experimental therapy for Retinitis Pigmentosa

Zheng Qin Yin
Southwest Hospital / Southwest Eye Hospital, Third Military Medical
University, Chongqing, 400038, China.

Abstract

Retinitis Pigmentosa is one of the leading causes of blindness worldwide and lacks effective clinical treatment. Stem cell-based therapy offers a novel experimental therapeutic approach, based on the strategy that transplanted progenitor cells could replace damaged photoreceptor cells. However, it is still unknown what is the optimal time to choose for targeting the host tissue during the progression of the degeneration, the characteristics and potential capacities in different stem cells, whether stem cells differentiate into functional daughter cells, and the degree to which host retinal function can be restored.

We have used Royal College of Surgeons (RCS) rats as a suitable model of retinitis pigmentosa and light induced photorecptor damage in minipigs to study the effectiveness of cell transplant therapies and the functional capcity of the retina. Initially, whole-cell patch clamp studies showed three action potential discharge patterns of retinal ganglion cells (RGCs) in RCS rats: single, transient, and sustained firing. The main discharge pattern was single firing between postnatal weeks 1 and 2 (P1-2W), followed later by transient and sustained firing patterns. However, during later stages of retinal degeneration at P7-8W, 26.7% RGCs lack action potentials in RCS rats, and this proportion had increased (63.2% of RGCs) by P9-12W. This suggested functional RGCs were maintained in the early stages of retinal degeneration, but this functional parameter was lost during retinal degeneration, even though morphological differences are not apparent. Cultured stem cells from embryonic rat retina differentiated and produced action potentials in vitro showing that the maturation of electrophysiological properties of presumptive RGCs occurs after at least 15 days under culture conditions. Knowledge of the timing of voltage-dependent ion channel development provides a time window stem cell funcitonal matureation that will help to improve success rate in transplantation protocols if functional recouvery is to be achieved. We found that, three types of stem cells (rat optic cup at embryonic day 12.5 (OC-RSCs), retinal stem cells from embryonic day 17 induced by BDNF (RSCs–BDNF) and rat bone marrow stromal cells (BMSCs)) were incorporated into the degenerating retina and differentiated into rhodopsin positive cells. Thus, all three stem cell types are suitable for retinal transplantation, although RSCs from different developmental stages have distinct proliferative capacities and differentiation potential. OC-RSCs are easier to passage, although a large number of E12.5 embryos are required. BMSCs are easier to obtain and can restore retinal function in RCS rats for up to two months after transplantation. The retinal transplantation in minipigs by neonatal pig retina or human fetal retina with an intact retinal pigment epithelium (RPE) was successful in 66.7% of the experiments. Twelve months follow up showed that xenografts transplantation had not resulted in any immunological rejection and thus was a safe technique. After the human fetal retina transplantation, the grafts survived and retained characteristics of progenitor precursor cells, such as Chx10 labeling. Multifocal electroretinography (mfERG) showed improvement of central posterior retinal function from the 1st to 8th month after transplantation. Müller cells are an integral and important glial component in the normal function of the retina and form an vital part of the regenertive process. Immunocytochemistry showed that Müller cells express retinal progenitor cell markers during chronic retina degeneration. After RSC transplantation, Müller cells were seen to differentiate into photoreceptors within and nearby the grafted area. This suggests that Müller cells have the potential to re-enter the cell cycle and can differentiate into host photoreceptor cells thus restoring lost retinal components. Further studies are needed to determine how to maintain the progenitor potential of Müller cells and how RCS transplants may augment this process of restoring cells, especially photoreceptors, to the damaged retina. These studies may help to understand how host retinal function can be restored with these combined techniques.

Introduction

There are few effective clinical treatments for retinal degenerative diseases such as retinitis pigmentosa (RP), a disease which affects an estimated 1.5 million individuals worldwide (Arai et al. 2004), and age-related macular degeneration, which is a leading cause of blindness in older individuals (Congdon et al. 2004). A variety of experimental therapies are under investigation aimed at repairing or rescuing impaired vision (Maclaren and Pearson 2007; Sieving et al. 2006; Maguire et al. 2008), including gene therapy and retinal transplantation. However, gene therapy was halted due to the difficulty of finding key target genes in the enormous number of RP-related genes. In addition, gene therapy can be only used in the early stage of RP. The limitations of gene therapy made the recent prospect of retinal transplantation more attractive. Various cells, tissues and devices have been investigated in retinal transplantation, including photoreceptor cells, retinal pigment epithelial (RPE) cells, embryonic or neural stem cells, bone marrow-derived stem cells, retinal stem/progenitor cells, fetal neuroretina (with or without RPE), and retinal prostheses (Maclaren and Pearson 2007; Inoue et al. 2007; Wang et al. 2008; Jensen and Rizzo 2006; MacLaren et al. 2006). However, there are still many points that need clarification and some of these are detailed below. Firstly, what is the most suitable time period during host degeneration for sub-retinal implantation, in order to produce the best functional rescue? Secondly, what are the characteristics and potential rescuing capacities of different donor cells? Thirdly, whether donor cells can differentiate into functional daughter cells with appropriate electrophysiological functions? Last but not least, how to restore host retinal function following sub-retinal implantation in RP? In our search for a possible clinical treatment strategy for RP, we studied these questions in a retinal degeneration model using Royal College of Surgeons (RCS) rats and light-induced retinal degeneration minipigs. The data is present in the following five parts.

Part I: Surviving Ganglion Cells - The Guide for Retinal Degeneration Stem Cell Therapy

Retinal ganglion cells (RGC) process and convey visual information from the retina to higher visual centers in the brain. Previous work reported that even in the late stages of retinal degeneration 4.9% of photoreceptors and 29.7% of RGCs were still preserved morphologically (Humayun et al. 1999; Villegas-Perez et al. 1998; Yoshimura 2001). After the absence of visual input caused by photoreceptor death in the RP, RGCs may become dysfunctional but retain their morphological characteristics. This is a crucial factor for host retinal tissue / stem cell transplantation. Therefore, it is important to investigate the morphology and electrophysiological changes of RGCs during retinal degeneration (Figure 1).

RGC membrane properties change considerably during postnatal development in normal rats, these changes being due to self-differentiation, gene expression, synapse formation, and development of projection of visual information to higher centers, etc. In our study, we used whole-cell recording on retinal ganglion cells of RCS rats to investigate the intrinsic membrane properties of these cells (Figure 2A). To our knowledge, this is the first study to directly address the alterations of electrophysiological properties of ganglion cells in RCS rat retinal slices. In addition, electrophysiological properties were compared among RCS rats with and without retinal degeneration, and normal Long–Evans rats. Our results demonstrated that retinal ganglion cells of RCS rats had similar electrophysiological properties to those of normal rats during the first 1–6 weeks, including resting membrane potential, input resistance, and AP (Figure 2B). There were three kinds of AP in RGCs of RCS rats: single, transient, and sustained firing patterns. Before eye-opening, single spikes were the main pattern. According to its high resting membrane potential and input resistance, and low amplitude and frequency of AP, we infer that single spike is the prophase of ganglion cells. Over development, the ratio of discharge patterns changed, and transient and sustained firing became the main patterns. These results were also obtained from control and normal rats. It is known that retinal degeneration begins right after birth in RCS rats (Eisenfeld et al. 1985). No significant changes were found in discharge patterns of ganglion cells in RCS rats at the early stage of postnatal development (Figure 3). The main discharge pattern was single firing in postnatal ages P1-2W, followed later by transient and sustained firing. However, during the later stages of retinal degeneration (P7-8W), 26.7% of RGCs lacked proper action potentials in RCS rats, and the proportion increased to 63.2% at ages P9-12W.

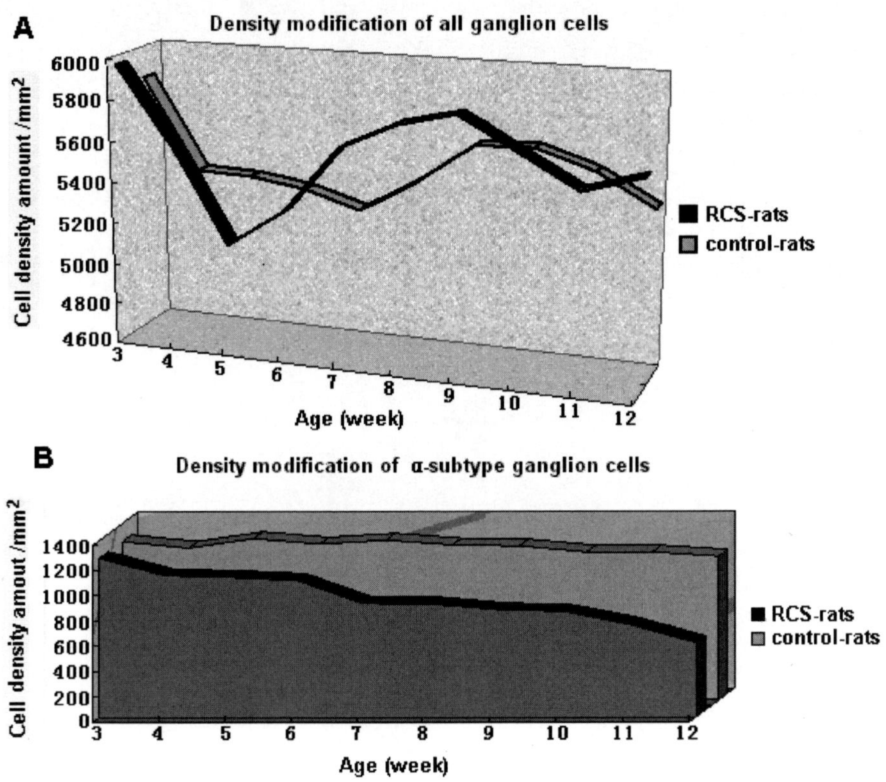

Fig. 1 The density modification of retinal ganglion cells during the retinal degeneration.

A. The density modification of all the retinal ganglion cells during the retinal degeneration. In the early stage of the degeneration, the density of the RCS have a temporal decreasing, significant less than the control, nevertheless similarity as the control in the later stage.

B. The density modification of α-retinal ganglion cells during the retinal degeneration.

The density of the RCS α-retinal ganglion cells kept on constant decreasing. From the Pn7 on, the density of the RCS retinal ganglion cells have a dramatic depletion that was significantly less than the control. (Chen-xing; et al. 2005)

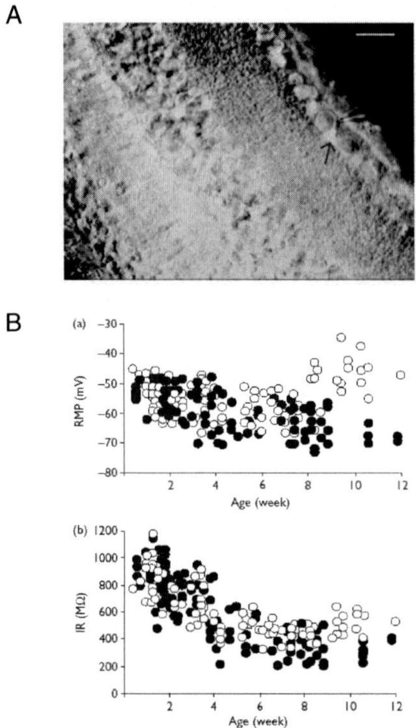

Figure2A Infrared microscope image of a rat retinal slice. A ganglion cell layer cell
was patched. The axonal process just below the soma (arrow) indicates that this cell is
probably a ganglion cell. Bar = 20 mm. Figure 2B (a) Comparison of resting membrane
potential (RMP) between Royal College of Surgeons (RCS) rats (hollow circles) and
normal (black circles) rats. (b) Comparison of input resistance (IR) between RCS
(hollowcircles) and normal (black circles) rats. (Chen et al, Neuroreport, 2005)

Beginning at P7-8W, in RCS rats, the ratio of discharge patterns of
ganglion cells changed, transient AP increasing and sustained AP decreasing
in frequency. After P9-12W, we detected slight changes on histological
examination of retinal ganglion cells in RCS rats. However, a dramatic change
was observed in the electrophysiological properties of ganglion cells: most of
the ganglion cells lacked discharge, even with high injection current. These
findings indicate that despite a lack of significant change in ganglion cell
morphology in RCS rats. In comparison, we found development appearing
constant and the sustained firing ratio increasing in normal and control rats
after eye-opening. It was known that the decrease in threshold and the rise in

amplitude of AP during development are closely related to the increase in density of sodium channels and decrease in threshold of activation of channels (Robinson and Wang 1998; Schmid and Guenther 1998; Skaliora et al. 1995). It has also been reported that frequency of firing is determined by the rate of recovery of sodium channels from inactivation. Sodium channels are inactivated following depolarization. In RCS rats, the resting membrane potential became more depolarized at a late developmental stage. It may

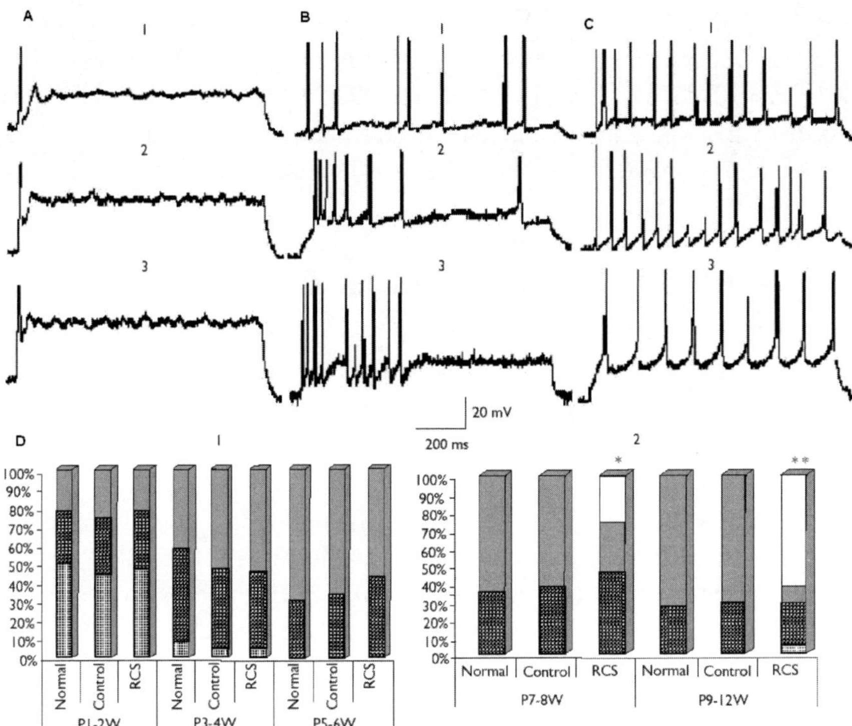

Figure 3A. Single spikes of RGCs (evoked by 60 pAdepolarizing current). (1)Normal rat, (2) control rat, and (3) Royal College of Surgeons (RCS) rat. B. Transient firing of ganglion cells in rats (evoked by 20 pA depolarizing current). (1) Normal rat, (2) control rat, and (3) RCS rat. C. Sustained firing of ganglion cells in rats (evoked by 20pA depolarizing current). (1) Normal rat, (2) control rat, and (3) RCS rat. D. The distribution of discharge patterns of ganglion cells in normal, control, and RCS rats: (1) normal (n=28,24,13), control (n=16,21,12), and RCS rats (n=19,26,14) from birth to P6W; (2) normal (n=14,11), control (n716,14), and RCS rats (n=15,19) during P7- 8W and P9-12W. *p<0.05 versus normal and control rats; **p<0.01 versus normal and control rats. (Chen et al, Neuroreport, 2005).

be that inactivation of sodium channels of ganglion cells increases and sodium channel intensity decreases with retinal degeneration. How this is related to the electrophysiological alterations that occur in ganglion cells of RCS rats remains to be determined (O'Brien et al. 2002). These results may aid determination of the optimal time for treatment and thus maximize treatment efficacy.

Summary: Our findings suggested that functional ganglion cells exist in RCS rats at early ages, but lose part of their function during the period of retinal degeneration, even though morphological differences are not yet apparent. Understanding the changes of electrophysiological characteristics during retinal degeneration in detail may help to develop the optimal time course for treating retinitis pigmentosa and particularly the appropriate time for cellular transplantation (Chen et al, Neuroreport, 2005).

Part II: Fifteen Days Ion Channel Maturation for Retinal Stem Cells - Benefit for thought in Future Transplantation Protocols

Besides RP host cells' function in part I, another key point for rescue RP is the characteristics of donor stem cells, which was reflected by not only antigen markers, but also cellular activities. The success of stem cell transplantation critically depends on whether the stem cells can differentiate into functional daughter cells. The neural stem cells that originate from the embryonic and adult central nervous system can be made to differentiate into neurons and neural glial cells and then labeled with specific antigens (Wegner and Stolt 2005). However, a criterion for neuronal differentiation based on the presence of neural antigens cannot satisfactorily predict neuronal function (Song et al. 2002). Thus, knowledge of functional criteria based on the presence of characteristic active membrane properties and functional synapses could play an important role (Reh 2002) in determining the efficacy of a therapeutic application.

Das et al (Das et al. 2005) reviewed the development of cell membrane properties of retinal stem/progenitors, including the differential expression of genes, physiological properties and the development of voltage dependent channels. However, data was presented for only the first few days after the induction of differentiation and while the development of potassium and sodium channels in these first few post-induction days was charted, it was intuited from the presence of outward and inward currents respectively, rather than from determining the effects of known channel blockers.

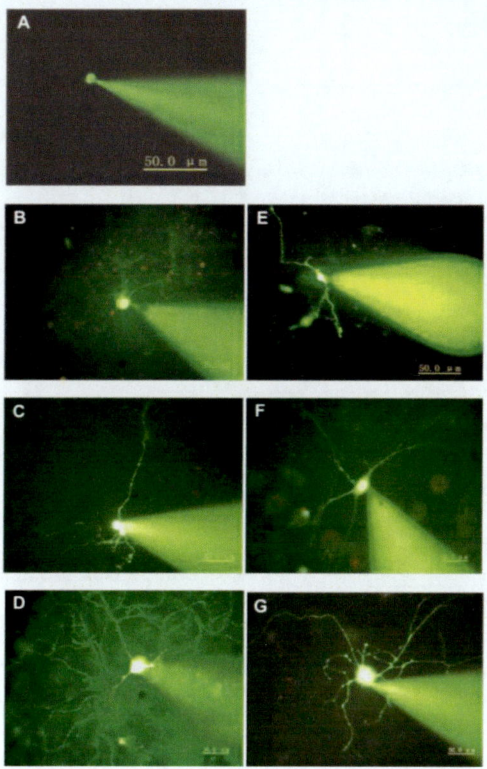

Figure 4. Differentiation of RSCs and the development of neuronal comparison group in culture. Cells were photographed following recordings and injection with Lucifer Yellow. Dendritic fields were larger and dendrites became thicker and longer with longer differentiation times (or time in culture). A, B, C, D: differentiated cells at DIV 0, 3, 7, 15 respectively from RSCs. E, F, G: comparison group neurons at days 3, 7, 15 in culture, respectively, scale bar = 50 μm. (Chen et al. IOVS, 2008).

The purpose of our study was to investigate the development of electrophysiological properties of rat RSCs derived from embryonic day 17, using whole-cell patch-clamp recording, following the induction of differentiation *in vitro* (DIV). We have used patch clamp techniques to confirm that RSCs express electrophysiological characteristics typical of differentiated retinal neurons and have determined their time course of development in culture. These results were compared to recordings from cultured retinal neurons. The data demonstrate the value of whole cell patch clamp recording in providing information on the developmental state of ion channels and neuronal function not available through anatomical techniques.

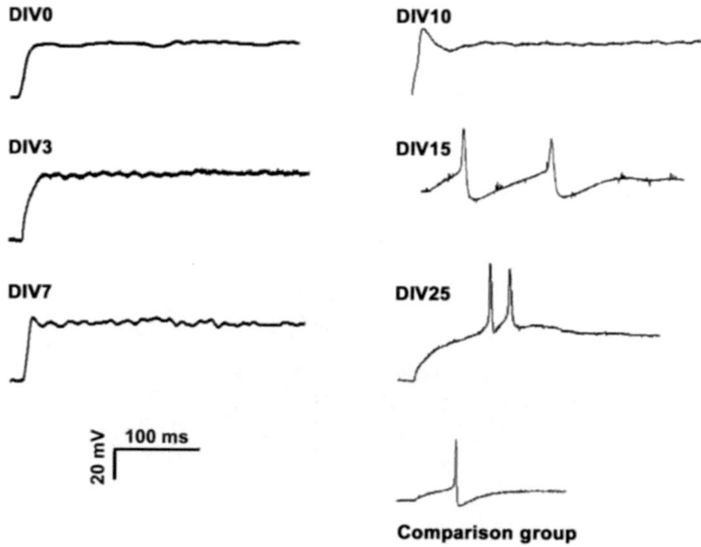

Figure 5. Differentiated stem cells can generate action potentials. Responses are shown to a 1000 ms 80 pA intracellular current pulse during current-clamped recordings from RSCs at different stages of DIV. Evoked APs could not be reliably generated in the cells before DIV10. At DIV10, a broad but shallow single evoked action potential could be recorded. By DIV 25 these APs resembled those in the comparison group and had a relatively mature firing pattern. (Chen et al. IOVS, 2008).

Previously, we (Chen et al. 2007), see also (Das et al. 2005) have systematically labeled cells with neuronal antigens or, as in the present study, used Lucifer Yellow injections to visualize dendritic cell morphology (Figure 4). However, these methods give no indication of the actual functional status of the labeled cells. Although one may argue that these cells are in the process of developing into mature neurons, many cultured or transplanted cells do not complete their development, and neuronal precursors and cell lines differ widely with respect to their capacity for maturation (Hales and Tyndale 1994; Sucher et al. 1993). Because of this a more stringent standard for neuronal identification has been proposed based on the identification of functional neuronal characteristics, such as electrical excitability (e.g. action potentials), and the ability to communicate information with other neurons via synapses. Thus, it is important to use techniques that establish the stage of functional maturity during differentiation and that can be applied when evaluating the clinical usefulness of successfully differentiated cultures as potential transplant material.

We evoked apparently mature APs when RSC differentiation had proceeded beyond DIV15 (Figure 5). In our cultures, APs are reliably evoked by day 10, albeit later than that reported by Das et al. (Das et al. 2005), who studied RSCs for 6 days following induction, compared to 25 days in this study, thus demonstrating that cultured RSCs harvested from embryonic rats can produce APs *in vitro*. However, spontaneous APs were not apparent until DIV 25 – at which stage they were indistinguishable from cultured retinal neurons (Figure 6).

The present results show that the neuron-like cells induced to differentiate from RSCs developed active electrophysiological features including inward sodium currents and outward potassium currents. Importantly, APs could be both induced and develop spontaneously. These latter cells exhibiting spontaneous APs are most likely retinal ganglion cells. During the process of stem cell differentiation, voltage-dependent ion channels gradually developed in a time dependent manner and ultimately support mature AP firing similar to that observed in the cultured postnatal cells. Distinct voltage-dependent currents emerged during different stages of stem cell development. This is similar to results recorded from cultured bone marrow stem cells, for which the gradual maturation of physiological parameters and antigen expression were concomitant (Kohyama et al. 2001; Warren and Jones 1997). Full maturation of K^+ and Ca^+ channels seemed to occur after 14 to 28 days in culture and is roughly in agreement with the present findings that the appearance of Na+ channels (DIV7) and their maturation at ~ DIV15 does not occur until after antigen expression (unpublished data). Our data also showed a significant correlation between channel and AP maturity and length of time in culture. Physiological recording from mouse thalamic cells in slice preparations have also noted the significant correlation between the size of the AP and postnatal age (Warren and Jones 1997). This time dependent feature may be a useful criteria for classifying the functional stage of maturity for cultured cells, particularly as considerable morphological variation was encountered in the differentiated cells.

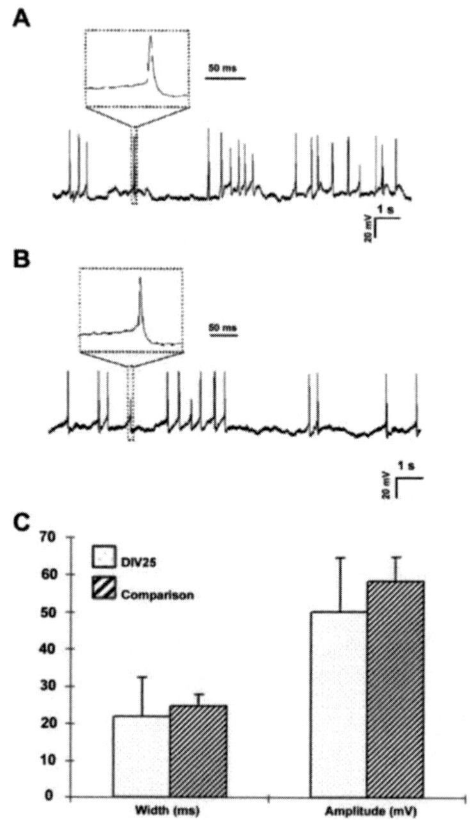

Figure 6. Differentiated stem cells can generate spontaneous action potentials.
Spontaneous APs occurred in RSCs at DIV25 (A), which were similar to those seen on
Day 7 in the comparison group (B). There are no significant differences between the
two groups in terms of wave width and amplitude (C). (Chen et al. IOVS, 2008).

Interestingly, during development we found a mixed population of TTX-
sensitive and TTX-insensitive cells (Figure 7). A similar finding was reported
by Wu et al. (Wu and Pan 2004), where Na+ channels were expressed in
different types of dorsal root ganglion (DRG) neurons. That study provides
complementary evidence that there were distinct differences in the expression
levels of TTX-S and TTX-R Na^+ channels between IB4-negative and IB4-
positive small-diameter DRG neurons. This difference in the density of TTX-
R Na^+ channels is responsible for the distinct membrane properties of these
two types of nociceptive neurons. This suggests that all RSCs develop Na^+
channels at the same differentiation time; however, the density and maturity of

the channels differs between cell types, thus leading to the differing electrophysiological properties of the channels. Previous work has shown that there are several types or classes of rat RGCs and that these cell classes differ in their maturation during early postnatal life (Perry and Walker 1980; Yamasaki and Ramoa 1993). This could suggest a delay in the saturation of the density of TTX-sensitive channels or a developmental insensitivity of individual channels to TTX. However, this latter question could not be resolved with the whole-cell patch clamp method. Similar findings were reported by Sun et al (Sun et al. 2005) relating to differentiating neural stem–like cells derived from the nonhematopoietic blood fraction of the human umbilical cord. Further work is necessary to unravel the developmental differences between these sodium channels and their effects on the development of cell morphology and function, including their affect on the evoked action potential arising from the two neural-like cells types containing differing amounts of TTX sensitive and insensitive Na^+ channels.

A question remains as to why there is expression of Na^+ channels at DIV7, but APs can not be evoked. We suspect that it is related to properties of immature Na^+ channels at some differentiation stages, and that only a sufficient density of mature Na^+ channels at the axon hillock can support evoked APs. During the development of rat retinal ganglion cells, the size and complexity of the dendritic trees were found to increase rapidly during an initial stage of development lasting from late fetal life until approximately postnatal day12 (Perry and Walker 1980; Yamasaki and Ramoa 1993), which is consistent with the time-course of morphological and physiological maturation at DIV15. Given the more mature starting point of RGCs from the postnatal day 1 (PND1) comparison group, the earlier appearance of K^+, Na^+ channels and APs in these neurons is consistent with the normal development of RGCs. Prior to eye-opening, waves of correlated AP firing spread across the RGC layer in response to Ca^+ flux, and this occurs before the functional maturation of the photoreceptors (Shatz 1996); these waves of spontaneous APs appear to be crucial for the early topographic organization of connections within the thalamus and cortex.

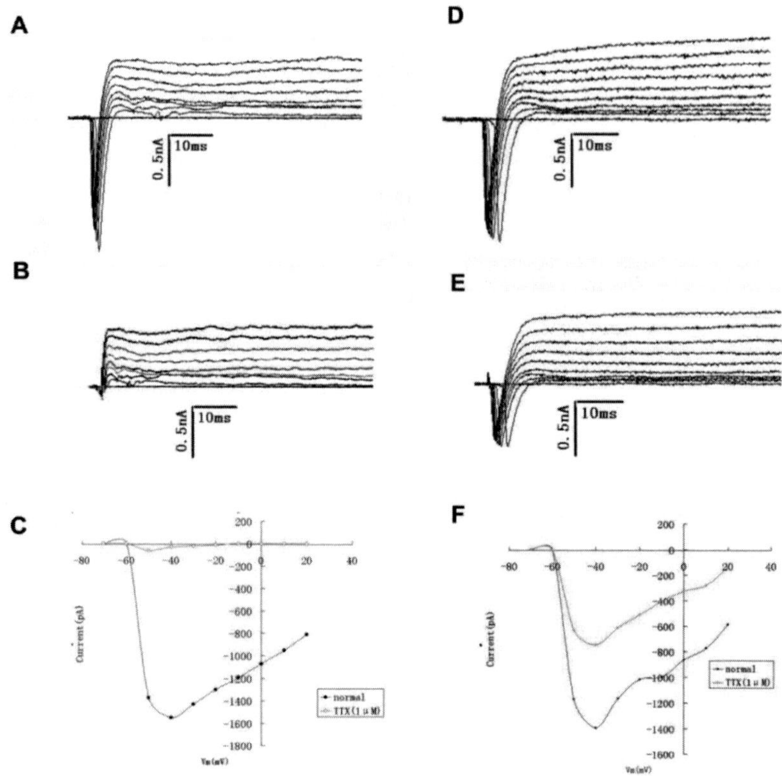

Figure 7. (A, D): Voltage-dependent sodium currents (I_{Na+}) could be recorded on DIV7 following induction of RSCs. Inward I_{Na+} was present in differentiated RSCs from DIV7 onwards: Sodium currents could be recorded in a voltage clamp configuration (holding potential -70 mV, voltage step from -80 to +100 mV, 20 mV/step). (B): TTX (1 μM) blocked Na^+ currents. (C): I/V curves of Na^+ currents without (●) and with 1 μM TTX (○). The currents were effectively blocked by TTX. (E, F): An example of a cell which was only partially blocked by 1 μM TTX (○). (Chen et al. IOVS, 2008).

Successful stem cell transplantation for degenerative retinal disorders depends upon a deep understanding of the characteristics of the stem cell (Djojosubroto and Arsenijevic 2008; Lu et al. 2008; Pellegrini et al. 2007). Our results suggest that functional maturation (i.e. APs) is not achieved until at least 15 in days in culture and RSCs, when differentiated to 25 days, can also develop spontaneous APs similar to that seen in the comparison group. The suitability of these cells for transplantation and their viability for integration within a host retina will require further detailed study.

Summary: Patch clamp electrophysiology of RSCs at various stages of differentiation is able to provide detailed timing data regarding the expression of various ion channels that may be critical for the correct synaptic connections to be made, eventually subserving functional visual perception. Oriented induction *in vitro* may be necessary before cell transplantation (MacLaren et al. 2006); and access to the electrophysiological function of induced RSCs should assist assessment of the suitability of the RSCs (Chen et al. IOVS, 2008).

Part III: Three Types of Stem Cells and their Subretinal Transplantation

After we know the RSCs has similar electrical excitability (e.g. action potentials) like neurons, the next step is to investigated detailed characteristics and rescuing capacities of different stem cells in retinal transplantation. In our laboratory, three types of stem cells (rat optic cup at embryonic day 12.5 (OC-RSCs), retinal stem cells embryonic day 17 induced by BDNF (RSCs-BDNF) and rat bone marrow stromal cells (BMSCs) pretreated with bFGF were cultured and transplanted into subretinal space of RCS rats. We found that these three kinds of cells were incorporated into the degenerated retina, differentiated into rhodopsin positive cells and restore the function of degenerative retina in RCS rat respectively.

1. Optic-Cup-Derived Retinal Stem Cells (OC-RSCs): Cell Cultures from the Rat Optic Cup at Embryonic Day 12.5

In retinogenesis, the tailbud stage is of special interest, because RSCs commence differentiation after this period. There is no retinal cell differentiation at the tailbud stage (embryonic day (ED) 11.5-12.5 in rat); RGCs are only generated later at ED13 in the rat (Zhao et al., 1995). Therefore, all cells in the optic cup at the tailbud stage are stem cells. Moreover, a major proliferation of optic cup cells in retinogenesis occurs between the time of the optic cup formation and the appearance of RGCs, causing thickening of the inner layer (Levine and Green, 2004). Thus, we hypothesized that it should be easier to produce well-purified RSCs with a high proliferative capacity from the optic cup at the tailbud stage and that this kind of stem cell could give rise to all major cell types of the retina. However, the information regarding the innate proliferative behavior and phenotypic potential of stem cells at this developmental stage remains unknown.

In our experiment, Thy1.1 protein was not detected at the tailbud stage (ED12.5) and this suggests that differentiated retinal cells are not yet present in the optic cup at ED12.5. Thus, we conclude that the cells in the optic cup at ED12.5 are all RSCs and should be amenable to enrichment through culture procedures. So, we isolated cells from the Long Evans rat optic cup at embryonic day 12.5 (tailbud stage), analyzed the characteristics of the cells. In vitro, most cells isolated from the optic cup at ED12.5 proliferated and formed neurospheres for at least eight passages and the colony-forming cells express the retinal progenitor marker CHX10 and Pax6. Presumptive retinal specific cell types were produced by the colony-forming cells after serum induction, as depicted by the expression of markers such as Thy1.1, GFAP, MAP2, PKCα and rhodopsin (Figure 1). The data indicated that these colony-forming cells are indeed retinal stem cells. According to their particular embryonic stage of origin, we named these colony-forming cells "optic-cup-derived retinal stem cells" (OC-RSCs). OC-RSCs grew either as monolayers or as neurospheres in the presence of bFGF. Our results suggest that the monolayer growth is a fundamental growth property of OC-RSCs in vitro. This property enabled us easily to characterize these cells immunocytochemically. In addition, OC-RSCs can be easily dissociated to single cell suspensions when grown as a monolayer making FACS analysis feasible, as well as cell suspensions used in transplantation injections. OC-RSCs produced retinal specific cells after the addition of serum to the medium, but the differentiation potential was affected by serum concentration. However, FBS is a common supplement for cell culture, as well as an inductor of stem cell differentiation (Das et al., 2005a), therefore, the effect of FBS on RSC differentiation should be taken into consideration, when designing future experiments.

We found that OC-RSCs are easily enriched to 92% by three passages, have normal diploid karyotype and exhibited no obvious differences in proliferative rate during eight passages (doubling time: 36 h) (Figure 2). This suggests that well-purified RSCs with high proliferative capacity can be easily obtained from ED12.5 embryos by just passaging the cells. Given the high proliferative capacity of OC-RSCs, we attribute the easy enrichment by passage to their growth dominance in culture. A major proliferative stage of optic cup retinogenesis occurs between the time of optic cup formation and the appearance of RGCs, causing thickening of the inner retinal layer (Chacko et al., 2000; Coles et al., 2004; Yang et al., 2002). This suggests that well-purified RSCs with a high proliferative capacity can be obtained from developing retina at this stage, during which extensive proliferation of RSCs occurs in the optic cup before initiation of retinal ganglion cell development. We have shown that OC-RSCs not only maintain a high proliferative rate and purity after at least 8 passages, but also maintain a normal diploid karyotype. These results suggest that a normal and sufficient number of OC-RSCs can be obtained from cultures on passages 3-8 which are suitable for transplantation. In order to verify that the neurogenic vs. gliogenic properties were similar in vitro and after transplantation, we transfected the OC-RSCs with the EGFP-plasmid after passage 3 and then transplanted the cells into the subretinal space of Royal College of Surgeons (RCS) rats, an animal model of retinal degeneration. OC-RSCs were found incorporated into the degenerated retina and differentiated into rhodopsin positive cells (Figure 3). These results demonstrate that survival of OC-RSCs after subretinal transplantation can occur and these cells can express a rhodopsin phenotype and be integrated into the degenerated host retina. This suggests OC-RSCs are suitable for retinal repair.

Thus, as an easily and well-purifed stem cell population with a high proliferative capacity and differentiation potential into photoreceptors after subretinal transplantation, OC-RSCs are suitable for retinal transplantation although RSCs from different developmental stages have distinct proliferative capacities and differentiation potential.

2. Retinal stem cells embryonic day 17 induced by BDNF (RSCs+BDNF)

RSCs-BDNF implanted subretinally were found incorporated into the degenerated retina and differentiated into rhodopsin positive cells (Figure 4). Thus, retinal stem cells embryonic day 17 induced by BDNF (RSCs+BDNF) are suitable for retinal transplantation although RSCs from different developmental stages have distinct proliferative capacities and differentiation potential (unpublished).

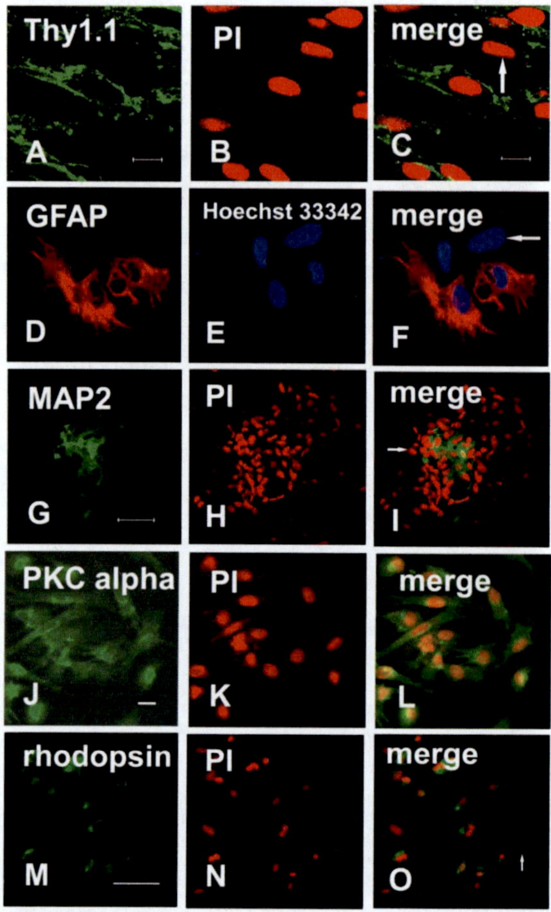

Figure 1. Differentiation of optic cup colony-forming cells. The differentiated optic cup colony-forming cells were stained with anti-Thy1.1 (A-C), anti-glial fibrillary acidic protein (*GFAP*) (D-F), anti-microtubule-associated protein (*MAP2*) (G-I), anti-protein kinase C alpha (*PKCα*) (J-L), and anti-rhodopsin (M-O). A subset of cells showed plasma membrane staining for Thy1.1 (A, *green*), and nuclear staining for PI (B, *red*). Note in C (*merge, arrow*) not all cells are double labeled. Cells stained for cytoskeletal GFAP (D, *red*) and nuclear staining for Hoechst 33342 (E, *blue*), showed that not all cells are GFAP positive (F, *merge, arrow*). A subset of cells showed cytoplasmic staining for MAP2 (G, *green*) or nuclear staining for PI (H, *red*), note the lack of double labeled cell in the merged photomicrograph (I, *arrow*). A subset of cells had cytoplasmic staining for PKCα (J, *green*), and nuclear staining for PI (K, *red*), (L, *merged*). Selective labeling of cells for rhodopsin (M, *green*) and nuclear staining for PI (N, *red*) shows that not all cells are opsin-positive (O, *merge, arrow*). *Bars* 20 μm (A-F, J-L), 50 μm (G-I, M-O) (Huang, et al: Cell Tissue Res, 2008)

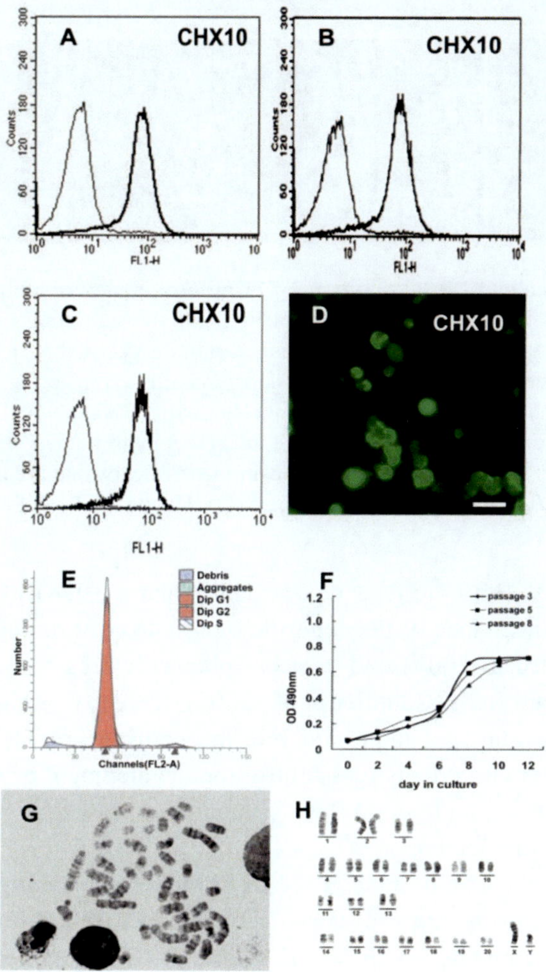

Figure 2. Purification and proliferative properties of OC-RSCs. A-C Flow cytometry results indicate that the percentage of CHX10-positive cells at passage 3, 5, and 8, respectively, was about 92%. (*horizontal axis* relative fluorescence, *vertical axis* cell counts). Compare the antibody-associated labeling (*right peak*) and isotype controls (*left peak*). D Smear of the CHX10-positive cells prior to flow cytometry, *Bar* 20 μm. E Cell cycle profile. Approximately 91.5% of the cells were in the G0/G1 phase (*Dip diploid*). F Proliferative activity is shown for passage 3, 5, and 8 cells in vitro, as detected by 3-(4, 5-dimethyl-thiazolyl-2)-2, 5-diphenyl tetrazolium bromide (*MTT*) assay and optical density measurement (*OD*). G Metaphase plate of culture during the eighth passage. H Karyotype of culture during the eighth passage (Huang, et al: Cell Tissue Res, 2008).

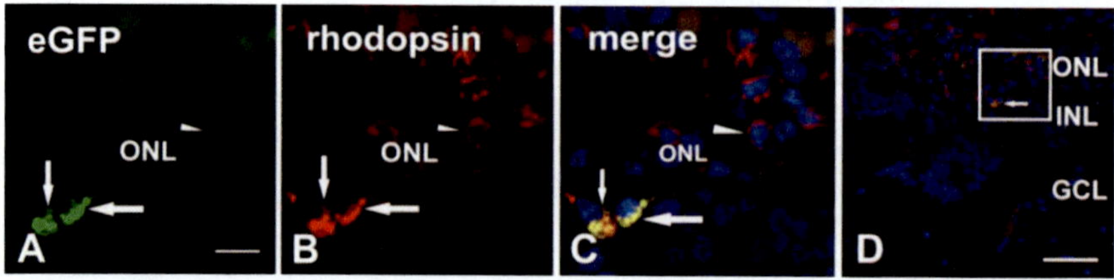

Figure 3. Transfected OC-RSCs in vivo. A-D Confocal images of recipient retina 4 weeks after eGFP-labeled cells were transplanted into the subretinal space of RCS rat. B, C Confocal images at high and low magnification, respectively, show examples of both eGFP-positive (*eGFP*, *green*) and rhodopsin-positive (*red*) cells (*arrow, arrowhead*) that had migrated to the outer nuclear layer (ONL). Not all rhodopsin-positive cells were labeled with eGFP. Note in D (*INL* inner nuclear layer, *GCL* ganglion cell layer) that a number of rhodopsin-positive cells that are not labeled with eGFP (*arrowhead*). Bars 10 μm (A-C), 50 μm (D) (Huang, et al: Cell Tissue Res, 2008).

In the retina, Brain-derived neurotrophic factor (BDNF) can support the survival and maintenance of the dendritic morphology of retinal ganglion cells (Weber and Harman 2008) and protects photoreceptors from the damaging effects of constant light (Gauthier et al., 2005). Recently, it has been reported that BDNF also plays an important role in dendritic growth in response to enriched visual environments that control the development of retinal circuitry (Landi et al., 2007; Landi et al., 2007). In addition, researchers found that, in the rat, BDNF can effectively

One of the most important goals for retina transplantation is to protect visual function during the process of retinal degeneration. We investigated whether BDNF combined with retinal stem cell (RSC) transplantation could provide a better restoration of visual function in degenerating retinas compared to previous approaches to the problem.

Retinal stem cells were derived from embryonic day 17 Long-Evans rats and pre-labeled with fluorescence pigment-DiI prior to transplant procedures. RCS rats received injections of retinal stem cells, stem cells+BDNF, phosphate buffered saline or BNDF alone (n = 3 eyes for each procedure). At 1, 2 and 3 months after transplantation, the outer nuclear layer thickness measured and the electroretinogram (ERG) were assessed.

We found that photoreceptor cell bodies are located in ONL of retina, therefore, measuring ONL thickness can indicate enhance cell survival and may represent the protection of the host retina (Fujieda and Sasaki 2008). We found both RSCs eyes and RSCs + BDNF eyes had thicker ONL layers compared to PBS and BDNF injected eyesat each time point and thus suggesting that the rate of photoreceptor degeneration and cell death is slowed down to some degree. The eyes receiving retinal stem cell and stem cell+BDNF transplants showed better photoreceptor maintenance than the other groups at all time points. Recent research has shown that exogenously applied BDNF can activate neuroprotective signaling pathways such as ERK1/2 and Akt and can upregulate endogenous production of BDNF by Müller cells in the mouse retina (Azadi et al., 2007). Others have demonstrated that BDNF and its receptor TrkB play a significant role in the regulation of neuronal growth, survival and synapse formation in the central nervous system and in the retina (Loeliger et al., 2008; Pinnock and Herbert 2008; Vissio et al., 2008; Xuan et al., 2008). Furthermore, BDNF-TrkB signaling regulated the maturational formation of new branches in ON-ganglion cells and controls cell-specific, experience-dependent remodeling of neuronal structures in the visual system (Liu et al., 2007; Grishanin et al., 2008; Marler et al., 2008).

One and two month after retina transplantation, the amplitudes of rod-ERG and Max-ERG b waves were significantly higher the eyes with RSCs and RSCs +BDNF group ($P < 0.01$) compare with BDNF,PBS and untreated group, however, this difference was not seen at three months post transplantation. BDNF treatment alone group (without transplanted cells) had no effect when compared to buffer injections (Figure 5). The present results indicate that BDNF can enhance the efficacy of the retinal stem cell transplantation in treating retinal degenerative disease for two months to delay the retinal function damage. These results was supported by Rosemarle et al (2005) in which they used the animal model of light induced photoreceptor degeneration rat and transplanted adenovirus mediated gene delivery of BDNF of Müller cells in vitreous.

Although RSCs+BDNF and RSCs transplants show a better maintenance of the ERG and ONL thickness than PBS and BDNF injections over the first two months albeit diminished, the enhancement due to RSCs+BDNF transplants was only apparent in the first month after the operation. We suggest that effects of the BDNF are limited due to diminished concentration of BDNF following transplantation. We figure that BDNF combined cell transplantation could get a better vision function restoration at first month after transplantation because of BDNF can help graft cells get a better survival rate. Or may be BDNF related signal pathway participate into synapse

 Zheng Qin Yin

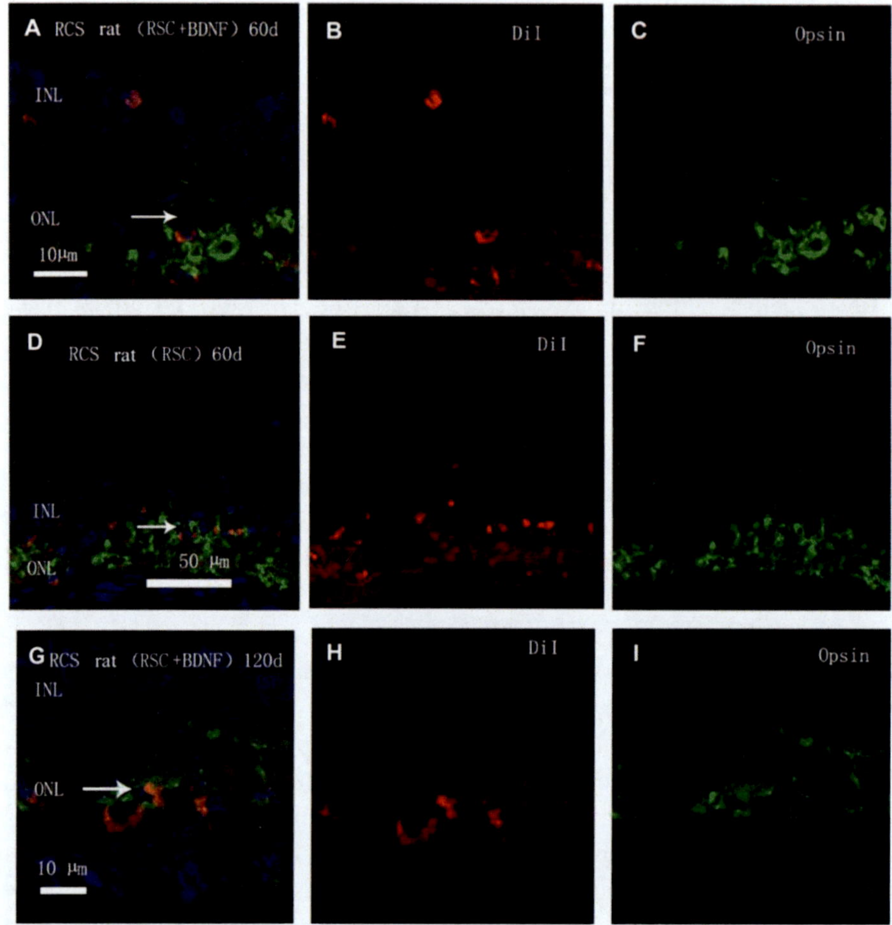

Figure 4 RSCs differentiated into Opsin positive cells. A-C RCS rat (RSCs + BDNF), 60 days post-transplantation. D-F RCS rat (RSCs), 60 days post-transplantation. G-I RCS rat (RSCs + BDNF), 120 days post-transplantation. Figure 4 Confocal images show examples of both DiI-positive (DiI, *red*) and Opsin-positive (*green*) cells (*arrow*) that had migrated to the outer nuclear layer (ONL). Bars 10 μm (A-C, G-I), 50 μm (D-F) (Unpublished data) minimize the retinal toxicity resulting from photodynamic therapy (Paskowitz et al., 2007).

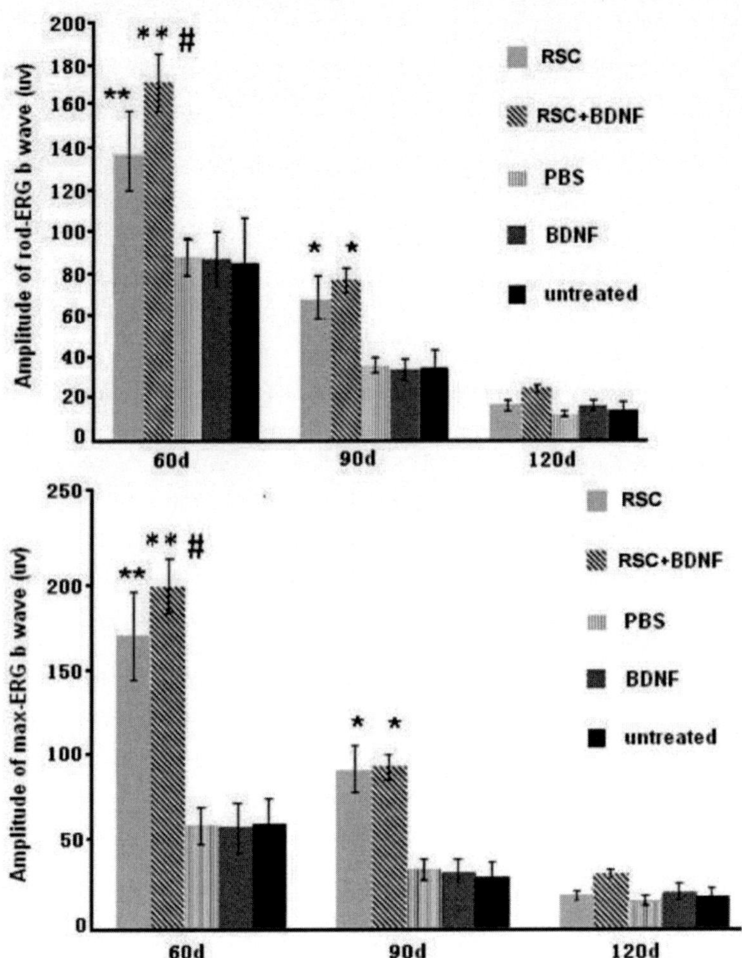

Figure 5. ERG amplitude measurements after transplantation. One month after transplantation, eyes receiving either RSCs or RSCs+BDNF transplants retained better ERG responses compared to eyes receiving PBS or BDNF injections (P < 0.01; bars represent the SEM). RSCs+BDNF eyes had significantly higher amplitude rod-ERG b (151 ± 31.5 μv vs. 137 ± 35.3 μv, P < 0.01, n = 3) and Max-ERG b waves (203.5 ± 27.4 μv vs. 174 ± 33.4 μv, P < 0.01) compared to RSCs eyes. At 2 months after transplantation, eyes receiving either RSCs or RSCs+BDNF transplants retained better ERG responses than PBS or BDNF, injected eyes P<0.01). However, there is no difference between RSCs or RSCs+BDNF eyes with respect to wave amplitude. At 3 months after transplantation, no differences were seen between groups. (Unpublished data).

formation and host retina circuitry. In the future, we will give the recipients multiple injections of exogenous BDNF to determine if a maintained concentration of BDNF is required to prolong the beneficial effects of RSCs transplantation, and obtaining a sufficient number of suitable donor cells still poses a significant problem for effective therapy.

3. Rat Bone Marrow Stromal Cells (BMSCs) Pretreated with bFGF

BMSCs implanted subretinally were found incorporated into the degenerated retina and differentiated into rhodopsin positive cells after subretinal transplantation.

Obtaining a sufficient number of suitable donor cells still poses a significant problem for effective stem cell therapy. The most promising stem cells available are bone marrow stromal cells (BMSCs). These cells offer distinct advantages by having autologous immunological characteristics and they are also relatively easy to isolate and to increase the cell numbers. A number of studies have shown that multipotent BMSCs can differentiate into osteoblasts, adipocytes, cardiac muscle cells as well as differentiating into neural lineages in vivo and in vitro. Yet recent controversy surrounds the mechanism of BMSC differentiation. Despite these concerns, however, BMSC differentiation into neuronal lines presents interesting new possibilities for generating sufficient BMSC-derived retinal neurons in vitro for effective transplant therapies.

We found that BMSCs can express retinal phenotypic markers in response to bFGF induction or retinal co-culture in vitro; however, there are significant differences in the proportion of cells expressing the various markers typical of a retinal neuronal cell population. Their data suggest that bFGF induction is superior to retinal co-cultures in inducing larger numbers of BMSCs to express neuronal phenotypes with short induction times, and a few cells stain positive for Thy1.1 than for opsin after bFGF induction. In the bFGF induction protocol, the expression of opsin (a photoreceptor marker) was only observed on day 1 and not in later cultures (Figure 6).

In our study, the labeled un-induced BMSCs (BMSCs) or bFGF induced cell mixtures (BMSCs+ bFGF) composed of BMSCs were transplanted into subretinal space in RCS-P+ (RCS) and RCS-rdy-P+ (normal rats). Survival, migration, differentiation and rescue effects of transplanted cells in the host retinal were evaluated at different time points.

Following transplantation into the subretinal space in RCS and normal rats, both BMSCs which was un-induced and induced- BMSCs which was cell mixtures with composed of phenotypically differentiated neurons and retinal neurons derived from BMSCs cultures survived for 3 months post-transplantation. The BMSCs had reached the GCL after 2 months post-transplantation in RCS rats, and were rarely seen in the GCL of normal rats after 3 months post transplantation. At all time points examined, the spread of BMSCs+ bFGF was significantly larger than that of BMSCs in both retina of the RCS and normal rats (Figure7A). The number of surviving cells in the RCS rat retina was significantly higher compared to transplants in the normal rat retina (P<0.05). Thus, transplanted cells had a greater capacity to survive in degenerating retine compared to normal retina. In addition, the survival rate of BMSCs+ bFGF in RCS or normal rat retina was significantly higher than that of BMSCs (P<0.05, P<0.01)(Figure7B). Differentiation in vivo showed that BMSC+ bFGF expressed Thy1.1 and GFAP in RCS rats, as well as BMSCs expressed Thy1.1 , opsin , **PKCα and GFAP in RCS rats, but only** GFAP in normal rats.

At one postoperative month the latency and amplitude of the Rod-ERG b wave showed significantly more recovery in transplanted animals compared to sham operated animals (P<0.05). A significant increase in the amplitude of the Max-ERG b wave was also observed 1 and 2 months post-transplantation (P<0.05). However, by 3 months the improvement in the Rod-ERG and Max-ERG b wave latency and amplitude had disappeared (P>0.05). Un-induced and BMSCs + bFGF made no significant difference (P>0.05) to photoreceptor rescue and flash-ERG function (Figure 7C, D).

BMSCs + bFGF containing phenotypic differentiated cells have stronger survival and migration abilities, and can rescue degeneration of photoreceptors and partly improve visual function in RCS rats after transplantation for 1 and 2 months but it has less differentiation compare with BMSCs. It provides a new direction for clinical transplantation in the future to further optimize the BMSCs, obtain an ideal method for transplantation and improve visual function.

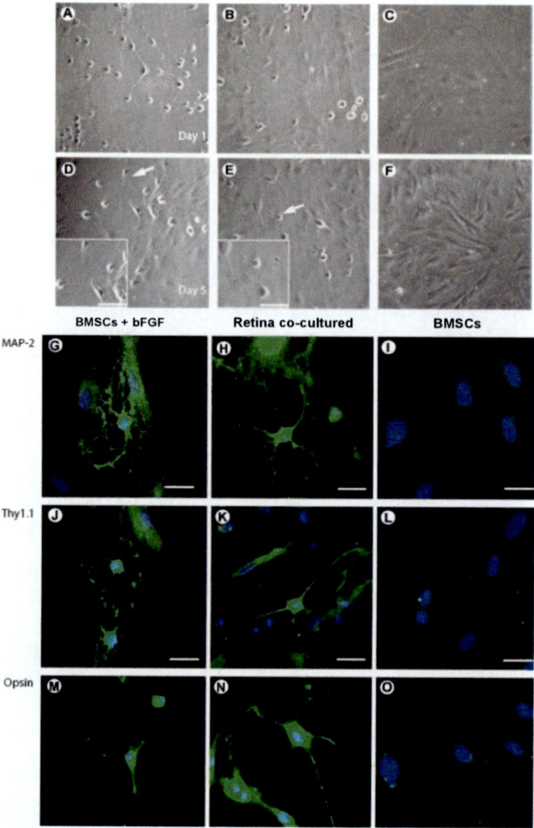

Figure 6. Phase contrast photomicrographs of bFGF induced and controls on days 1 and 3 after induction, and expression of retinal neuronal markers in both induction protocols. BMSCs + bFGF progressively changed from a spindle-shape into neuronal-like cells after 1 (A), and 3 days (D) induction. B, E BMSCs co-cultured with retinal cells exhibited a neuronal-like appearance with long processes. The processes on these cells developed more branches, some of which contacted the processes of other cells (see also J, K). C, F The BMSCs in the control group remained spindle-shaped during the induction period. The BMSCs + bFGF stained positively for MAP-2 (G), Thy1.1 (J) and opsin (M) at day 1. The BMSCs co-cultured with retinal cells from PN0–3 rats stained positively for MAP-2 (H), Thy1.1 (K) and opsin (N) at day 5. The cells in the control group were not stained with MAP-2 (I), Thy1.1 (L) and opsin (O). DAPI was used to counterstain cell nuclei. Scale bar in A-F = 100 µm; scale bar in G , H , J , K , M , N = 20 µ m; scale bar in I , L , O= 10 µm. (Liu, et al: Ophthalmic Research, 2009).

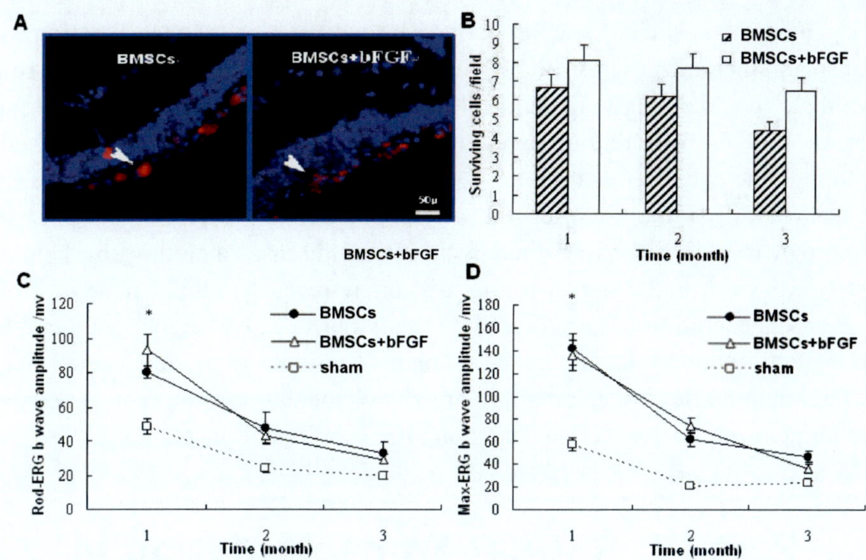

Figure 7. BMSCs + bFGF/BMSCs in vivo, Rod-ERG b wave amplitude and Max-ERG b wave amplitude. A 1 month after BMSCs + bFGF and BMSCs were transplanted into the subretinal space of RCS rat, confocal images of recipient retina show many cells were labeled with Dil. B After 3 months post-transplantation in RCS rats, the number of BMSCs + bFGF was significantly higher than that of un-induced BMSCs (P<0.05). * (P<0.05). C Rod-ERG b wave amplitude after 1, 2, and 3 months post-transplantation in RCS rats, compared with sham operation. * (P<0.05). D Max-ERG b wave amplitude after 1, 2, and 3 months post-transplantation in RCS rats, compared with sham operation. * (P<0.05). Bar 10 μm (Unpublished data).

Summary: Three types of stem cells (rat optic cup at embryonic day 12.5 (OC-RSCs), retinal stem cells embryonic day 17 pretreated with BDNF (RSCs–BDNF) and rat bone marrow stromal cells (BMSCs) can restore RCS rats' **retinal function for** 2 months after transplantation, thus are suitable for retinal transplantation although RSCs from different developmental stages have distinct proliferative capacities and differentiation potential. As an easily and well-purified stem cell population with a high proliferative capacity and differentiation potential into photoreceptors after subretinal transplantation, OC-RSCs provide a useful tool for the study of RSC differentiation and transplantation research, especially offer greater potential for manipulating differentiation into specific retinal phenotypes, but mainly in laboratory since a large number of E12.5 embryos are required. BMSCs are easier to obtain, and differentiate into retinal cell types presents interesting new possibilities for generating sufficient BMSC-derived retinal neurons in vitro for effective transplant therapies. Thus BMSC is one of the most promising stem cells available for the study of clinical cell-transplantation research in retinal disease, but the differentiation rate to retinal cell type needs improvement. Although the enhancement due to RSCs+BDNF transplants was only apparent in the first two month after the operation, cellular factors will play an important role in cell-based therapy in retinal disease, including by helping graft cells get a better survival rate, and/or by rescuing retinal neurons from further degeneration. Therefore, with high purity, easy to be got, and be pretreated with cell factors for high survival rate and determined differentiation after transplantation, are key elements for stem cells to achieve the purpose that restore retinal function after subretinal transplantation.

Part IV: Retinal Transplantation in Minipigs by Neonatal Piggy Retina or Human Fetal Retina with Retinal Pigment Epithelium

The investigation of donor stem cells for retina transplantation has covered photoreceptor cells, retinal pigment epithelial (RPE) cells, embryonic or neural stem cells, bone marrow-derived stem cells, retinal stem/progenitor cells and fetal neuroretina (with or without RPE) (Maclaren and Pearson 2007; Inoue et al. 2007; Wang et al. 2008; Jensen and Rizzo 2006; MacLaren et al. 2006). However, transplanting only the neuroretina or RPE has limited restorative capacity (Maclaren and Pearson 2007; Sakaguchi et al. 2004). On the other hand, fetal neuroretina with RPE is potentially more efficacious because it preserves an intact microenvironment or "stem cell niche" for the retinal stem/progenitor cells (Bendall et al. 2007; Raymond et al. 2006).

Previous reports using subretinal transplantation of fetal neuroretina with RPE showed a disorganized graft in mice (Aramant and Seiler 2002), and in human trials (Radtke et al. 2008) there was no improvement of visual function when tested by objective methods such as the multifocal electroretinogram (mfERG). However, the previous experiments used dispase to aid in tissue isolation, whereas, subsequent studies have shown that the enzyme may injure retinal ganglion cells and bipolar cells (Wang et al. 2004). Previously, we have shown that excimer laser is particularly useful for dissecting fetal tissue as it causes minimal damage (Chen et al. 2005) and therefore may be superior to dispase treatment.

A minipig model of light-induced retinal degeneration was reported in 1996 (Dureau et al. 1996), in which the outer nuclear layer was reduced by around 20% after exposure to high intensity white fluorescent light for one to three months. We used this model and excimer laser dissection to test whether a subretinal transplant of intact piggy or human fetal neuroretina with RPE will improve retinal function. We tested this using histological and electrophysiological techniques following transplantation.

1. Light Induced Retinal Degeneration in Minipigs

Three month old minipigs were used (from the Animal Institute of the Third Military Medical University, Guangxi Bama, China). In normal controls group, minipigs were exposed to 1000 lux daily light for 12 h. In light damaged group, minipigs were exposed for six months to 12 h per day of constant white light (400-700 nm) produced by neon tubes situated 1.5 m above the animals. The intensity at head level was measured as 2500 lux by a digital luxmeter.

A mfERG was recorded from each light-damaged minipig before and after light exposure (including control minipigs). Responses were measured using RETI scan (Roland Consult, Wiesbaden, Germany) connected to an ERG Jet gold contact lens electrode and a subdermal steel reference electrode 1 cm away from the lateral canthus (a steel subdermal ground electrode was placed between the eyes) (Figure1A). Each data set was generated as the average of eight consecutive runs, after which the 103 focal responses were divided into six concentric rings and an average waveform generated for each ring. The porcine mfERG trace has three peaks, Negative 1 (N1), Positive 1 (P1) and Negative 2 (N2), which were calculated according to the guidelines for basic mfERG (Marmor et al. 2003) (Figure . 1B & C). Light exposed minipigs that did not show a significant mfERG decrease were excluded.

After six months white light exposure (light-damage), the mfERGs of affected eyes showed a decrease in retinal function compared with normal eyes such that the amplitude density of the P1 wave significantly decreased in rings 1 - 4 (Figure . 1D), as well as the amplitude of the P1 wave in rings 1 - 6 (Figure . 1E). The N1 wave amplitude significantly decreased in rings 1 - 6 (data not shown). These changes in the N1 and P1 waves were more obvious at three and twelve months after light-damage. The latencies of the N1 and P1 waves were not significantly different (data not shown).

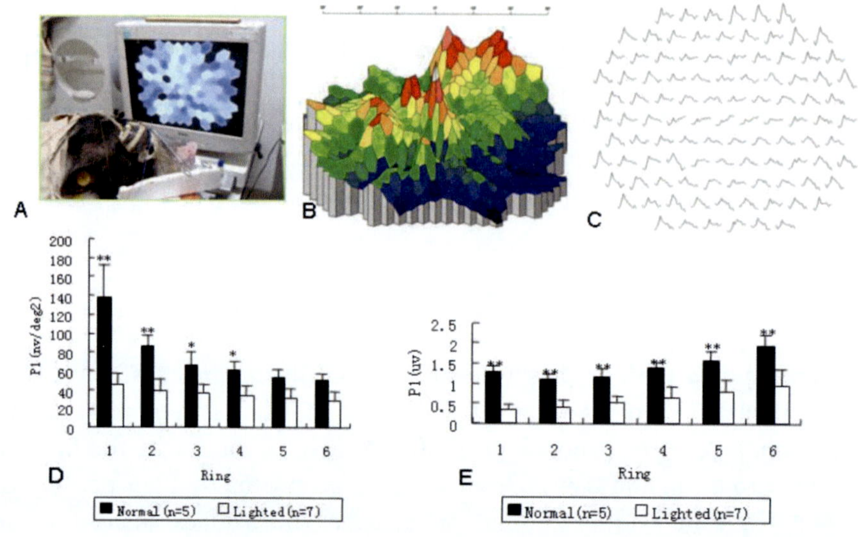

Figure 1. mfERG test on light induced retinal degeneration in minipigs. (A)Minipig was anesthesia and checked by RETI scan. (B and C)Light-damaged minipig showed flat waveform in posterior lighted area in three dimension map (B) and plots (C). (D and E) Statistic analysis showed decreased amplitude density (D) and amplitude (E)of the P1 wave in normal and light-damaged minipigs.(Unpublished data).

2. Retinal Transplantation in Minipigs by Neonatal Piggy Retina With RPE

Donor animals and recipient animals

Three postnatal day 1-5 minipigs, weighting 0.25 ~ 0.45kg, and 12 two month old minipigs weighting 3.0~4.2 kg were used for the donor and light-damaged recipients respectively. The eyes of the light-damaged minipigs were divided into 3 groups: I (n = 2 eyes) light-damaged eyes used to evaluate photoreceptor degeneration; II (n = 20 eyes) light-damaged eyes receiving retinal transplants, whose hosts were sacrificed by pentobarbital overdose 1, 2, 3, 4, 5 months after transplantation; III (n = 2 eyes) light-damaged eyes with sham operation whose hosts were sacrificed two months after the grafting operation.

Preparation of neonatal porcine neuroretinal grafts and transplantation

Eyes of 6 neonatal minipigs (1 to 5 days) postnatal age under general anesthesia thoroughly, The retina +RPE were dissected free of the choroid and sclera , and a 5 x 5 mm area involving the macular were removed and placed on a piece of 50% gelatin film (200 μm thick by 7.5 mm in diameter; Sigma, USA.). The tissue was placed with the choroid uppermost in 4°C Ames' solution and the choroid vaporized by a 193 nm excimer laser (Allegretto Wavetm Eye-Q, Germany) without damaging the RPE (Figure 2A). Another piece of gelatin film was then placed on the graft creating a sandwich. The sandwich was stored in 4°C Ames' solution until the pieces were loaded into a custom-made implantation tool prior to transplantation.

Twenty light-damaged eyes underwent subretinal transplantation of neonatal porcine retinal tissue by vitrectomy with a custom made siliconized glass cannula (China Patent CN200994858) (Figure2B). Sham operations were performed in 2 degeneration eyes.Months 1,2,3,4,5 after transplantation, the morphology was demonstrated by colour fundus photography, fundus fluorescence angiography (FFA) and histology, the retinal function was evaluated by mfERG.

In vivo and in vitro observation of the host retina and grafts

During In vivo observation, any superficial hemorrhages induced by the implant or sham procedure were absorbed within a short period of time. The position of the graft beds could be clearly seen in some retinas 1-2 months after transplantation as gray grafts((Figure 2C), but by five months graft position was not apparent. In the sham operated and 5 month post-transplantation retina, we only found retinochoriodal scars and achroma in the transplanted area. Fundus fluorescence angiography showed that there was some vessel leakage around the area of the transplants at between 1 and 3 months post transplantation, but there were no signs of rejection such as cystoid macular edema, and new vessel growth (Figure 2D). In vitro histology showed graft remained flat and connected with host 4 month post transplantation(Figure 2E).

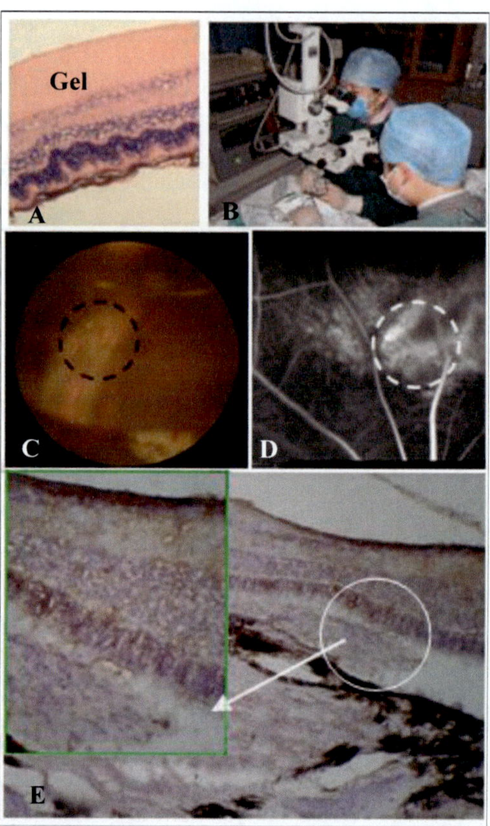

Figure 2. In vivo and in vitro observation of the host retina and grafts (A). **The graft's choroid was vaporized by a 193 nm excimer laser without damaging the RPE(Figure2A)** (B) minipigs underwent subretinal transplantation of neonatal porcine retinal tissue by vitrectomy (C). Fundus chromophotographs showed gray graft (black dot line)inside transplantation bed in host retina one month after grafting. (D).FFA showed an increase in the fluroscence around the graft area(white dot line) two month after grafting. (E) In vitro histology showed graft (white arrow) remained flat and connected with host 4 month post transplantation. (Unpublished data).

Host retinal function

mfERG of transplanted eye in same minipig(#5) in five months post transplantation showed that the amplitude of the P1 wave increased in ring 1 and 2, while the P1 wave in ring 3,4 and 5 decreased in 2nd month then increased from 3rd to 5th month post transplantation (Figure 3A). The amplitude of the N1 wave increased in ring 1, while the N1 wave in ring 2,3,4 and 5 decreased in 2nd month then increased from 3rd to 5th month post transplantation(Figure 3B).

3. Retinal Transplantation in Minipigs by Neonatal Human Fetal Retina with RPE Preparation of Fetal Graft of Neuroretina with RPE

Eyes from eight human fetuses 12 to 24 week in gestational age were obtained from the Eye Bank of the Third Military Medical University. All procedures adhered to the principles described in the protocol of Helsinki and were approved by the human ethics committee of the Southwest Hospital, Third Military Medical University. The full thickness of the choroid, retina and RPE of the donor eyes were dissected free from surrounding tissues and a 5 x 5 mm area involving the macular were removed and placed on a piece of 50% gelatin film (200 μm thick by 7.5 mm in diameter; Sigma, USA.). The choroid of tissue was vaporized by a 193 nm excimer laser and the fetal retina+RPE was sandwiched by gelatin using the same method in preparing neonatal porcine neuroretinal grafts above. The remaining tissue was kept in **Ames' solution for 2, 4, 6 and 8 h after the extraction** from the fetal retina, then digested by pancreatin, and stained with trypan blue. The percentages of viable cells (viability = live cell number/live cell number + dead cell number) were 95.5 ± 2.1% (n = 8), 85.0 ± 2.6% (n = 8), 76.5 ± 3.5% (n = 8), and 41.5 ± 4.8% (n = 8), respectively.

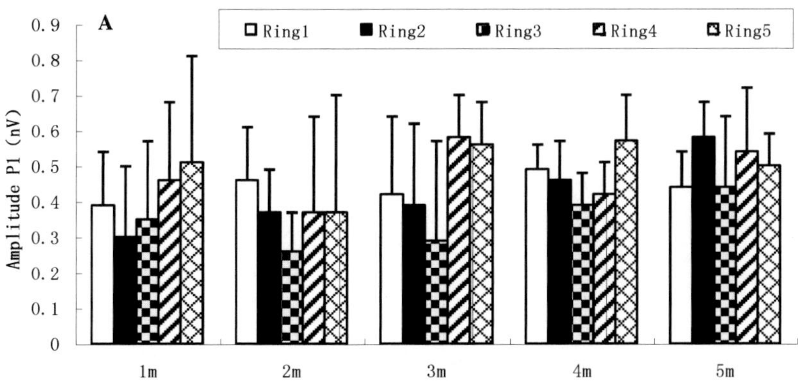

Figure 3 (Continued).

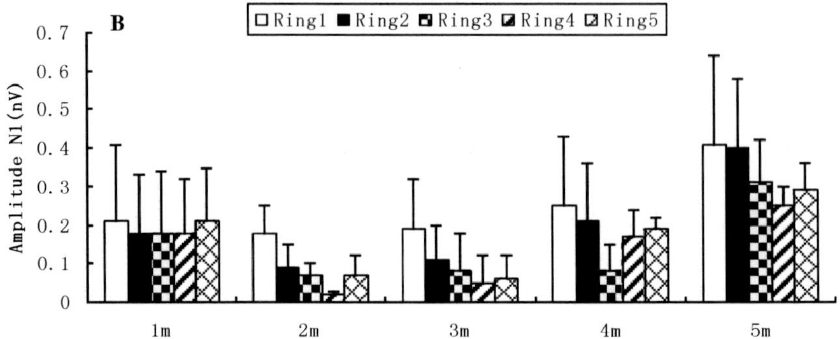

Figure 3. Comparison of amplitude of mfERG among 1,2,3 and 5months post-transplantation in light-damaged minipig (5#). (A) the amplitude of the P1 wave increased in ring 1 and 2, while the P1 wave in ring 3,4 and 5 decreased in 2nd month then increased from 3rd to 5th month post transplantation. (B) the amplitude of the N1 wave increased in ring 1, while the N1 wave in ring 2,3,4 and 5 decreased in 2nd month then increased from 3rd to 5th month post transplantation. (Unpublished data)

Host

Photoreceptor degeneration was induced by 2500 lux white light exposure for six months in 16 minipigs using method described above.

One normal control minipig received a subretinal fetal transplant and was killed immediately after the operation and the eye used for histology to assess the surgical effects. The 16 light-damaged minipigs were divided into three groups: Group 1 (n = 25 eyes) consisted of light-damaged hosts receiving retinal transplants with same method described above, then they were killed 1, 2, 3, 5, 8 or 12 months later by pentobarbital overdose. Group 2 (n = 3 eyes) were light-damaged animals with sham operations (a subretinal injection consisting of only Ames' media) and were killed 5 or 12 months postoperatively. Group 3 (n = 4 eyes) consisted of light-damaged animals without transplants that were killed 3 or 12 months after light damage and prepared for histology.Months 1,2,3,4,5 8 and 12 after transplantation, the morphology was demonstrated by colour fundus photography, fundus fluorescence angiography (FFA) and histology, the retinal function was evaluated by mfERG.

In vivo observation of grafts

Grafts were successfully inserted into the subretinal space of 25 light-damaged eyes (Group 1), of which 15 (60%) appeared normal over the 12 month experimental period (Table 2). Two eyes had corneal opacification resulting from exposure keratitis but subsequently recovered transparency. Three eyes had lens opacification (one of which included a focal retinal detachment) that developed into cataracts. Five eyes had retinal detachments due to focal retinotomy, three of which did not change, while the remaining two eyes displayed focal vitreal proliferation. These ten eyes (2 corneal exposure keratitis, 3 cataracts and 5 retinal detachments) were excluded from the study. Fundus fluorescence angiography showed no evidence of inflammation or edema in any of the eyes, indicating that immune rejection of the graft had not occurred.

Histology of graft

Figure 4A shows the characteristic position and orientation of a transplanted graft immediately after the operation. It is clear that the choriod has been almost completely removed from the graft tissue, while the neuroretina and RPE maintained a well laminated appearance and correct orientation within the host subretinal space.

Graft tissue was positively identified in the subretinal space in 10 out of the 15 eyes without complications. There were no signs of the supporting gel, nor was there evidence of necrosis and inflammation in the host retina, especially the host tissue around blood vessels where inflammatory cells (e.g. neutrophilic cells with lobulated or rod-shaped nuclei) usually appear (Figure . 4D insert).

One month after transplantation, the graft appeared as a non-laminated mass in the subretinal space. Note that in the example shown in Figure 4B there appear to be numerous tissue processes between the graft and the host retina. By the 2nd month the transplant appeared less dense and consisted of an accumulation of GFAP positive glia (Figure4C,) that appeared to be closely fused with the host tissue (see also Figure5A). By the 3rd (Figure . 4D), 5th (Figure . 4F,G, Figure . 5B,C), 8th (Figure . 4H) and 12th month (Figure . 4I) after transplantation, glial cells were the dominant cell type in the graft and some glial processes were present between the host and graft (Figure5B, C). Twelve months post- operation, both the host and grafttissue appear degenerative (Figure . 4I). All 10 eyes with histologically confirmed grafts had an anatomical relationship interposed between the graft and host tissue.

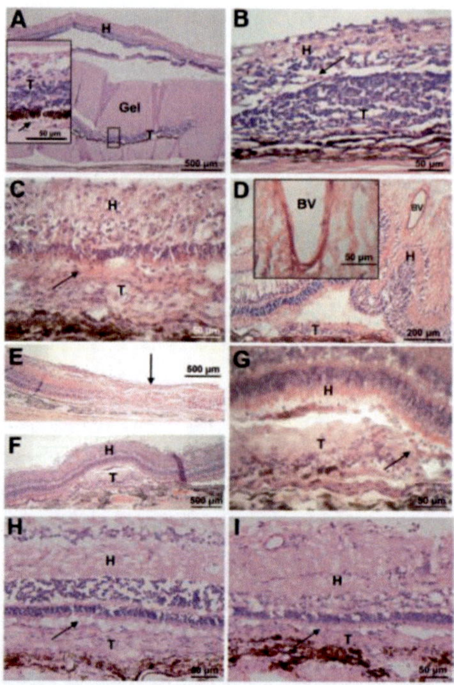

Figure 4. Hematoxylin and eosin staining of the host retina and graft implant. (A) The graft sandwich structure was transplanted with correct polarity into the subretinal space of a normal minipig. The retinal pigment epithelium (RPE) of the graft remained intact and the choroid (arrow) has been almost completely removed (see the high power insert; arrow indicates the residual choroid of the graft). H: host, T: transplant, Gel: 50% gel. (B) One month after implantation, graft number 11L appeared as a non-laminated mass in the subretinal space. . Note there appear to be numerous tissue processes (arrows) between the graft and the host retina. (C) Two months after grafting, glial cells (next to arrow, see also Figure .5A) accumulated at the graft site of animal 14R. (D), Although the shape of the host retina (10L) was disrupted three months after implantation, the retina maintained a laminated structure and there were no signs of necrosis or inflammation near blood vessels where inflammatory cells (e.g. neutrophilic cells with lobulated or rod-shaped nuclei) usually appear (BV; see the high power insert). (E) Five months after sham operation, retina 17R retained its laminated structure, although the sham insert site was sealed by glial tissue (arrow). (F, G) The graft in the other eye, 17L. There were some tissue processes between the graft and host retina (G, arrow). Note the graft has maintained some degree of lamination (G). (H) After eight months survival the graft in retina 9L, which contained many glial cells, had a number stainable material with the host retina (H, arrow). (I) After 12 months graft 2R contained largely glial cells, still had a number stainable material with the host retina (I, arrow). (Shi-ying et al, Current Eye Research, 2009).

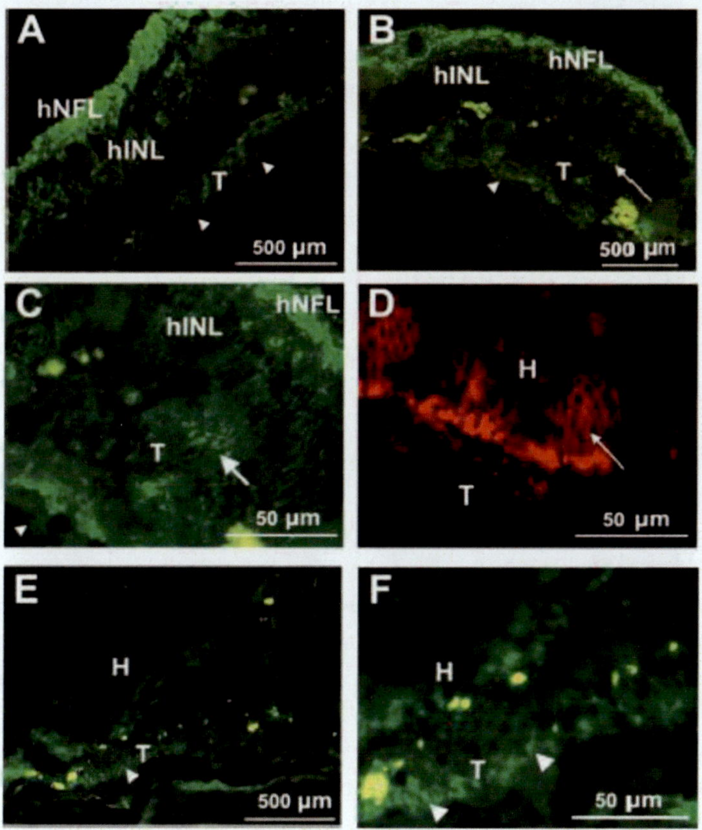

Figure 5. Immunofluorescent labeling of the host and graft tissue (cf. Figure . 4). (A) GFAP conjugated to fluorescein isothiocyanate-(FITC) shows the position of glial elements within the host nerve fiber layer (hNFL), host inner nuclear layer (hINL) and transplant (T) two months after light-damage (animal 14R; arrowheads show host RPE). (B, C) Five months after light-damage (animal 17L; arrowheads indicate the position of the host RPE) there were some glial processes or elements between the host and transplant (arrow). (D) Example of tissue immunostained with a Texas Red isothiocyanate (TRITC)-conjugated antibody for rhodopsin: animal 14R, two months after receiving a transplant. The transplant was rhodopsin negative, while the host retina showed labeling concentrated to the outer segments of the photoreceptors (arrows). (E, F) FITC conjugated Chx10 antibodies positively stained scattered profiles (arrowheads) in this graft three months after light-damage indicating the presence of retinal stem/progenitor cells. Labelling was not found in the host retina (animal 10L). H: host retina, T: transplant. hNFL: host nerve fiber layer, hIPL: host inner plexiform layer. (Shi-ying et al, Current Eye Research, 2009).

The rhodopsin-positive immuno labeling was found in the outer segment of host photoreceptors, but not in the graft by the 1st(data not show), 2nd (Figure .5 D), 3rd month (data not show) after transplantation. Chx10 positive cells (retinal progenitor cell marker) were found scattered within the graft (Figure .5E, F) at three months post-transplantation but were not present within the host retina.

Effect on host retinal function

In one minipig(#17), we compared the mfERGs of a grafted and sham operated eye in same sudject over a five month period (Figure . 6). In the right sham-operated eye (RS), the P1 wave amplitude density, P1 wave amplitude (P1RS) and N1 wave amplitude (N1RS) decreased compared with the eye containing the graft (left eye, LT). In contrast, in the left transplanted eye (LT), the mfERG showed that the P1 wave amplitude density and P1 wave amplitude (P1LT) in central retina (rings 1 and 2) substantially increased in the 1st, 3rd and 5th month, while in the paracentral retina (rings 3, 4, 5 and 6) the P1 wave amplitude density and P1 wave amplitude (P1LT), and the N1 wave amplitude (N1LT) increased in the 1st and 3rd month; note however, that the extent of the P1 wave amplitude increase is greater in rings 1 and 6.

The statistic mfERG data from all 15 eyes without surgical complications (i.e. eyes with (n = 10) and without (n =5) histologically verified grafts) after transplantation is summarized in Figure 8. The five eyes without an obvious graft presence were included because they also showed improvement in the mfERG. We attributed this improvement to the presence of the graft, which may either have escaped through the retinotomy hole and then been ultimately reabsorbed by the host or was missed during sectioning due to its small size. The eyes with sham operation showed no functional recovery. The P1 wave amplitude density within ring 1 and the P1 amplitude in rings 1 and 2 (central retina) increased compared with their pre-transplantation values (Figure . 8A, B). The N1 wave amplitude increased in both central (rings 1 and 2) and paracentral retina (rings 3-6) compared with pre-transplantation values (Figure . 8C). The latency of N1 and P1 waves did not show significant changes (data not shown). These mfERG changes were characterized by two peaks over eight months: the P1 and N1 wave amplitudes, and P1 wave amplitude density were enhanced in the 1st month after transplantation, maintained in the 2nd month, but subsequently significantly increased in the 3rd and 5th month, and remained until the 8th month. The mfERG values at 12 months are not included due to insufficient minipig numbers for statistical comparison.

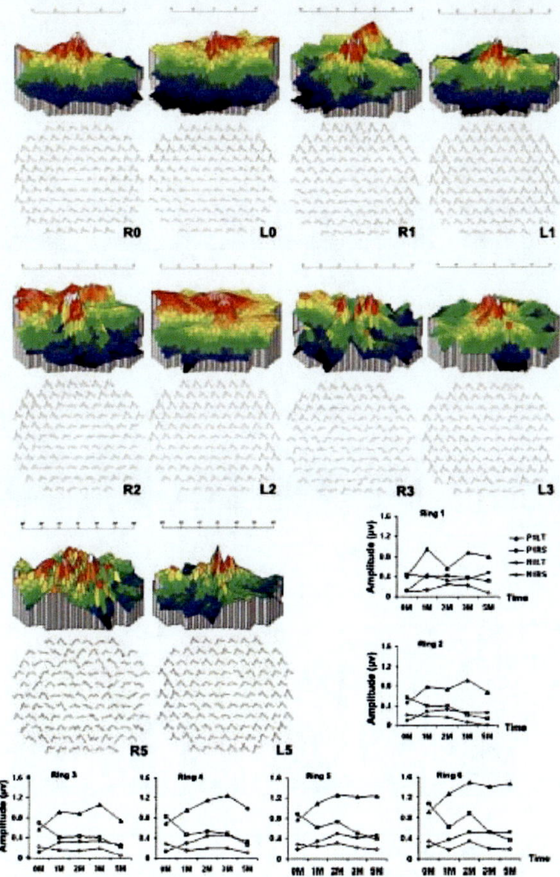

Figure 6. Comparison of mfERG amplitude and latency of P1 and N1 waves between the eye receiving the transplant (L: Left eye) and the sham operated eye (R: Right eye) in light-damaged minipig #17 (0-before operation, 1, 2, 3, and 5-months post-transplantation). The N1, P1 and N2 traces are plotted beneath the three dimensioned tomography. Note that the transplant does not occupy ring 1, the area centralis. The amplitudes of P1 and N1 wave for each ring are shown in line graph for easier comparison. The P1 wave *amplitude* (P1RS) and N1 wave amplitude (N1RS) in the right sham-operated eye decreased compared to its fellow eye containing the graft. In contrast to the sham operated eye, in the eye with the graft, the mfERG showed differences between central and paracentral retina; central retina (rings 1 and 2) showed that the P1 wave *amplitude density* and P1 wave *amplitude* in the left transplanted eye (P1LT) substantially increased in the 1st, 3rd and 5th month, while in the paracentral retina (rings 3, 4, 5 and 6) the P1 wave *amplitude density* and P1 wave *amplitude* (P1LT), and the N1 wave amplitude (N1LT) increased in the 1st and 3rd month; note, however, that the extent of the P1 wave *amplitude* density increase is higher in rings 1 and 6. (Shi-ying et al, Current Eye Research, 2009).

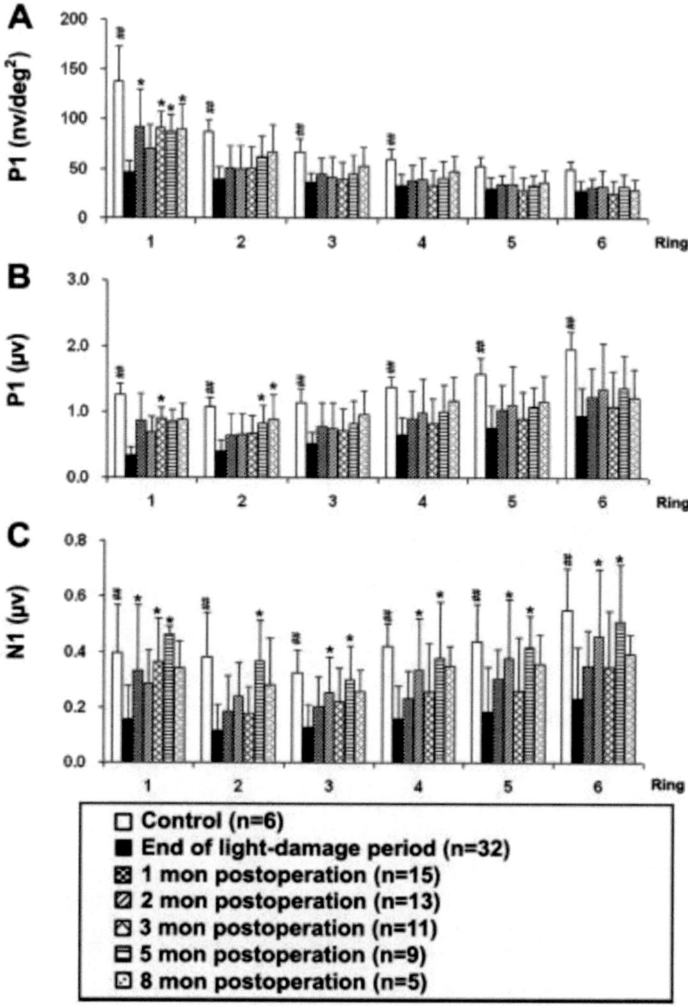

Figure 7. mfERG analysis of the P1 and N1 wave in the normal control (n = 6), at the end of light-damage period (n = 32) and in the light-damaged eyes with a graft after various survival times (n is shown with the graph legend). The P1 wave *amplitude density* within ring 1 and the *amplitude* in rings 1 and 2 increased, compared with their pre-transplantation values (A, B). The N1 wave amplitude increased in central (rings 1 and 2) and paracentral retina (rings 3-6) compared with pre-transplantation values (C). These changes were characterized by two peaks over eight months: 1st and 3rd to 5th month postoperation. ## $P < 0.05$: control eyes vs. eyes at the end of light-damage period. * $P < 0.05$ end eyes at the end of light-damage period vs. light-damaged eyes with transplants at 1, 2, 3, 5 and 8 months after surgery. (Shi-ying et al, Current Eye Research, 2009).

Summary

We formed a transplantation methods in large animal model which may be similar to future method used in clinical trial, and we examined the ability of the intact neonatal piggy and human fetal retina (neuroretina+RPE) to become incorporated into a degenerating retina, its fate after transplantation and its effect on host retinal function. Neonatal piggy and human fetal grafts maintained good viability after laser microablation and survived for 5 or 12 months in the light-damaged retina without signs of rejection. In addition, by using an objective functional test (mfERG) (Hood et al. 1998) we have shown retinal functional improvement not only in the transplanted area but also in the areas adjacent to the grafts. However, in this model of photoreceptor degeneration the fetal grafts preferentially adopted a glial cell fate and failed to differentiate into photoreceptors.

These observations collectively suggest that intact neonatal piggy or fetal neuroretina and RPE dissected by excimer laser can be safely sustained in a degenerating host retina, and maintains a largely glial cell population which may become activated and partially restores retinal function. We suggest that this functional restoration is due to the factors from the healthy retinal stem/progenitor cells and the stem cell niche in the intact graft, which maybe not achieved by pure cells transplantation.

Part V: Contribution of Müller cells before and after retinal stem cell transplantation

In Part IV, the large population of glial cells in the graft appeared to be associated with partially restoration of host retinal function and indicates that some unknown effects of glial cells may play an important role in functional recovery after transplantation. Many studies have recognized radial glial cells, which arise from neuroepithelial cells, as scaffolds for immature neurons migrating to the cortical plate during neurogenesis. While recent evidence suggests that the radial glia could also participate in neural regeneration and show multipotential characteristic of neural stem cells in adult mammalian CNS. With regard to the retina, which is a part of the CNS, it has been indicated that Müller cells are the radial glia of the neural retina. Recent studies have shown that they could behave as endogenous retinal progenitor cells and suggest their proliferative and regenerative potentials in vitro or in vivo, under certain special conditions.

Retinal precursors occur persistently in lower vertebrates such as fish and amphibian, which endows them with the ability to self- repair after retinal injuries. In adult mammals, it was previously thought that there were no retinal precursors in the retina. However, recent studies show that retinal precursors are found in different part of retina (Perron and Harris 2000), such as the retinal ciliary epithelium (Ahmad et al. 2000; Tropepe, 2000) and the pigmented epithelium of the iris (Asami et al. 2007; Haruta et al. 2001; Sun, 2006 #827). Some research has shown that retinal Müller cells in adult mammals also had the potential to become retinal precursors (Fischer and Reh 2001; Ooto et al. 2004; Osakada, 2007). To identify retinal precursors, some homodomains and transcription factors emerging at early developmental stages are used such as Chx10 (Vsx2) and Pax6. Chx10 has important effects on the development of the eyeball, and emerges initially in the optic vesicle, after Pax6. Combined with Pax6, Chx10 is expressed in retinal precursors during development of eye (Liu et al. 1994).

In lower vertebrates such as fish and amphibian, in vitro studies indicated that the cultured Müller cell could form neurosphere like structures, express Nestin- the marker of neuronal stem cells- and differentiate into multiple retinal neurons (Florian et al. 2008; Monnin et al. 2007; Nickerson et al. 2008). Müller cells may have the potential to de-differentiate in vivo into retinal precursor cells (Bernardos et al. 2007 Fausett, 2008 #696; Fausett et al. 2008; Fimbel et al. 2007; Thummel et al. 2008a; Thummel et al. 2008b). In mammalian retina, Müller cells normally can not re-enter the cell cycle, but have the ability to de-differentiate following some acute injuries such as NMDA induced RGC and amacrine cell death in mouse retina (Karl et al. 2008), MNU induced photoreceptor death in rats (Wan et al. 2008) and acute laser induced retinal injuries in mouse retina (Kohno et al. 2006). In these acute retinal injuries, Müller cells were found to re-enter the cell cycle and to de-differentiate into retinal precursors, amacrine cells, and photoreceptors to partially rescue the injured retina.

However, it is still unknown whether Müller cells might de-differentiate into retina progenitor cells in a rat model of chronic retinal degeneration with or without subretinal stem cell transplantation.

1. Müller cells de-differentiate into retinal precursors during the progress of retinal degeneration in RCS rats

To determine whether Müller cell de-differentiation happens during the progress of retinal degeneration in RCS rats we co-labeled Müller cells with Vimentin- a Müller cell specific marker- and Chx10- a retinal precursor markers. We found that at postnatal day 30 (30d) and 60d, some Müller cells showed positive staining for Chx10, which was not found in control group. The co-expression of Chx10 implies that Müller cells can de-differentiate into retinal precursors once the retinal degeneration begins, especially at progressing stage of retinal degeneration (Figure 1).

To identify the de-differentiation potential of Müller cells further, we co-cultured normal Müller cells (isolated from control rat retina) with a mixture of degenerating retinal cells obtained from RCS rats. The result showed that at 7 days after co-culture, the normal Müller cells also partially expressed Chx10, which strongly suggested that the de-differentiation of Müller cells can be induced by stimuli resulting from retinal degeneration (Fig. 5.2). Our hypothesis is that retinal degeneration acts like a chronic stimulating factor that continually stimulates the retina to express growth factors, thereby inducing Müller cells to undergo de-**differentiation and start the "self repair system".

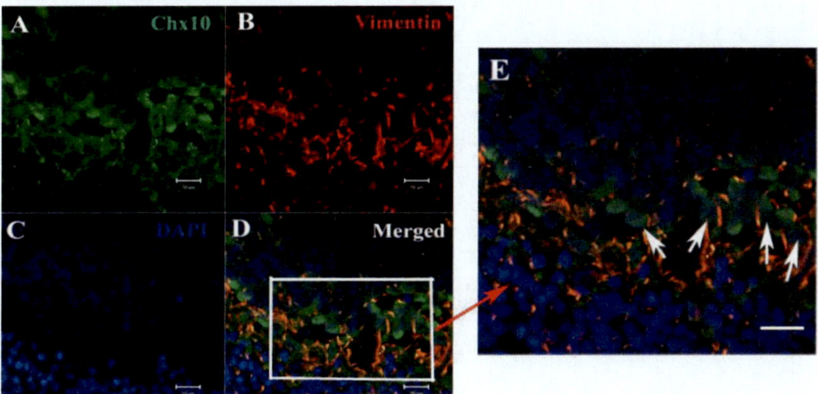

Figure 1. (A-D) At postnatal day 60 (60d) some Müller cells showed positive staining of Chx10 RCS rats. (E) In the inner nuclear layer, some vimentin positive cells showed Chx10 staining around the nucleus (short arrow). A: Chx10 staining (green);B: Vimentin staining (red); C: DAPI; D: merged. E: higher magnification of are in D. (A-D: scale bar = 20μm; E: scale bar = 10 μm).(unpublished data).

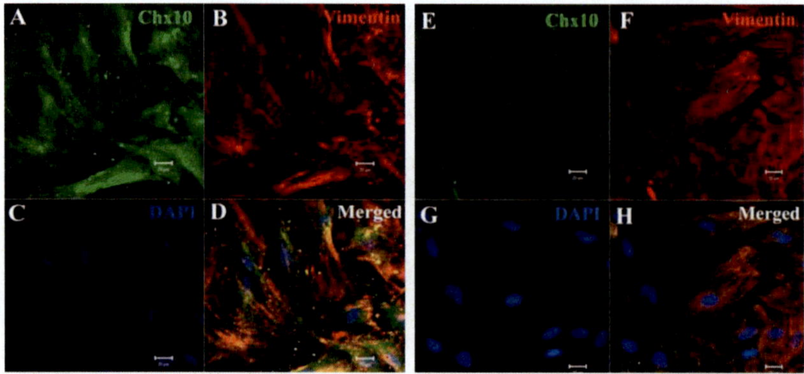

Figure 2. After 7 days co-culture, normal Müller cells partially expressed Chx10, which was not found in the control group (E-H; co-cultured with normal mixed retinal cells). A: Chx10 staining (green); B: Vimentin staining (red); C: DAPI; D: merged. (Scale bar = 20μm) (**unpublished data**).

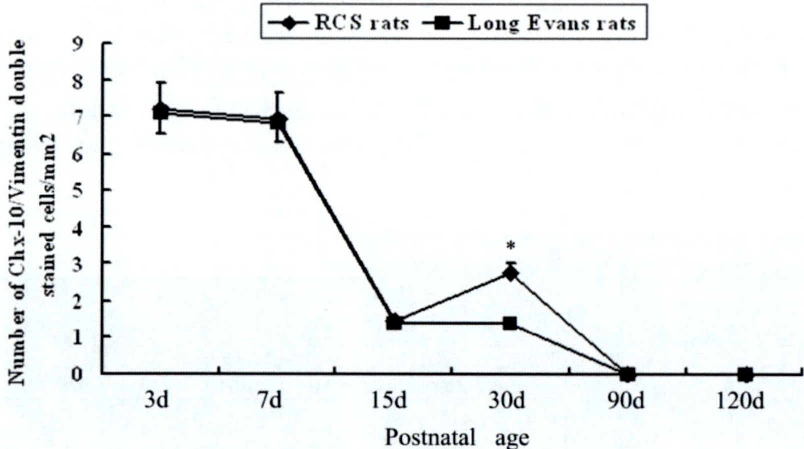

Figure 3. Changes of the number of Chx10/Vimentin double staining cells at the retinal margin at different postnatal ages in **RCS and Long Evan's rats**. *: P < 0.05, vs. Long-Evan's rats of the same age n = 6. (Qian Jian et al. Neuroscience Letter, 2009).

We assessed the active changes of Chx10 / Vimentin (1:500, Santa Cruz, Santa Cruz, CA) double staining with age in the center of retina of RCS rats and Long Evans rats prior to eye-opening to eye-opening (after 15d). Positive cells were counted per mm^2. We found that the number of the Chx10 / Vimentin double staining cells in the retina of RCS rats and Long Evan's rats decreased gradually from 3d to 15d. However, positive cells in RCS rats increased significantly at 30d ($p < 0.05$; $n = 6$), while no significant changes were observed in Long Evan's rats of the same age (Figure 3).

We have demonstrate that during the progression of retinal degeneration, the numbers of progenitor cells derived from Müller cells in RCS rats are significantly increased at 30d and 60d, then subsequently reduced at 90d. After eye-opening, the number of Chx10 / vimentin double labeled cells in RCS rats was significantly higher at 30d compared to Long Evan's rats, suggesting that during the development of retinal degeneration, the induced Müller cells potentially de-differentiated into progenitor cells; thus this time point is important for exploring retinal stem cell (RSC) activity.

2. Transplantation of retinal stem cells can promote de-differentiation of Müller cells in RCS rats

Rat RSCs were harvested from embryonic day 17 rat embryos, which were removed under sterile conditions from anesthetized pregnant Long Evans rats (Taconic, Hudson, NY). The subretinal space of RCS rats were injected on 30d, with either DiI prelabeled rat RSCs or PBS buffer. Animals were sacrificed on 60d, 90d and120d and the retinas stained with anti-Chx10 and vimentin. Firstly, we found that few DiI labeled graft cells still retained their progenitor cell characteristic after transplantation. CHx10 labeled Müller glia cells increased dramatically in RCS rats that received RSC transplants compared with controls (Figure 1). We also found some anti-recoverin positive staining- rod and cone photoreceptor anti-body- appeared in the inner nuclear layer (INL) and could be double labeled with vimentin on 60d, 90d and 120d (Figure 2) indicating that some of these Müller cells could co-express a photoreceptor cell marker..

More interestingly, we found that after RSC transplants, the number of dedifferentiated Müller cells in the non–operated area of the retina (nasal side) also increased (Figure 3). We counted the double labeled Chx10 and vimentin cells and found that 93.3±3% (60d), 89.9±3% (90d) and 91.9±3% (120d) of Chx10-positive cells co- expressed vimentin (Fig. 5.6) in RCS rats with RSCs, suggesting that after RCS rats received RSCs transplantation, the majority of newly appearing progenitors cells came from Müller cell de-differentiation although ~10% may come from other sources.

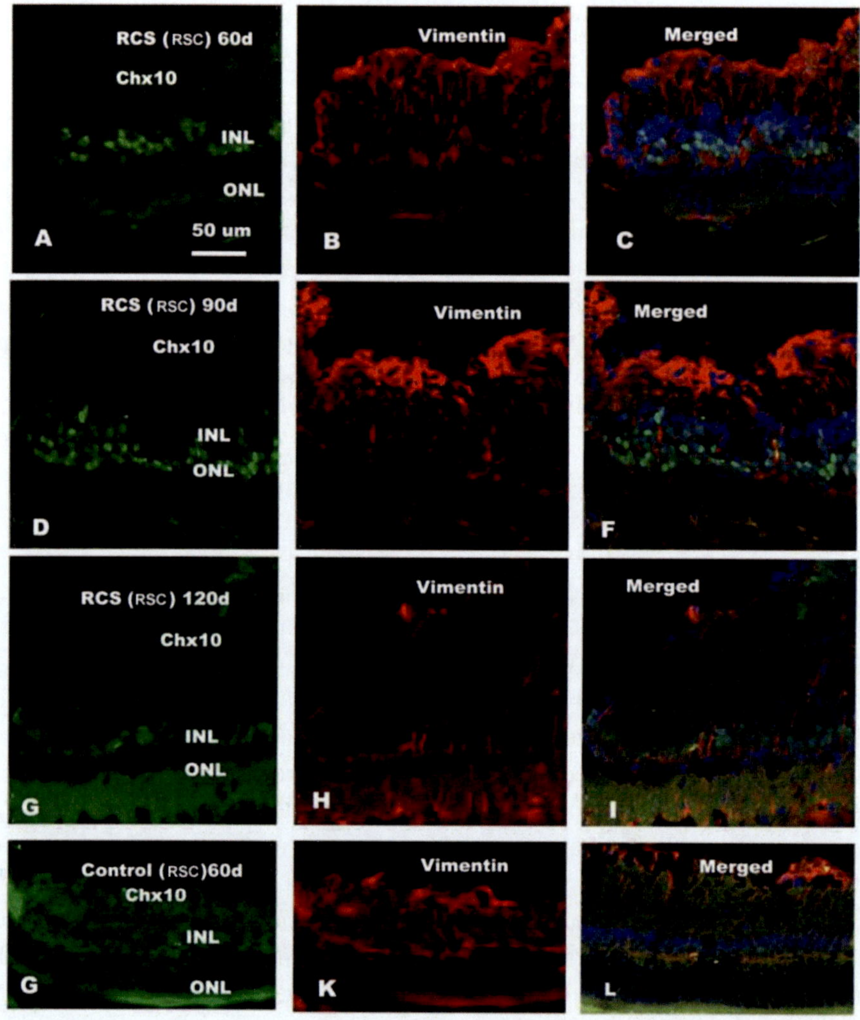

Figure 1. Transplantation of retinal stem cells (RSCs) induced Müller cells to de-differentiate. Retinal precursors were labeled by Chx10 (green). Müller cells were labeled by vimentin (red). A-C: Post transplantation 60d, D-F: 90d, G-I: 120d, J-L: Control RSC 60d.. scale bar = 50μm. (unpublished data).

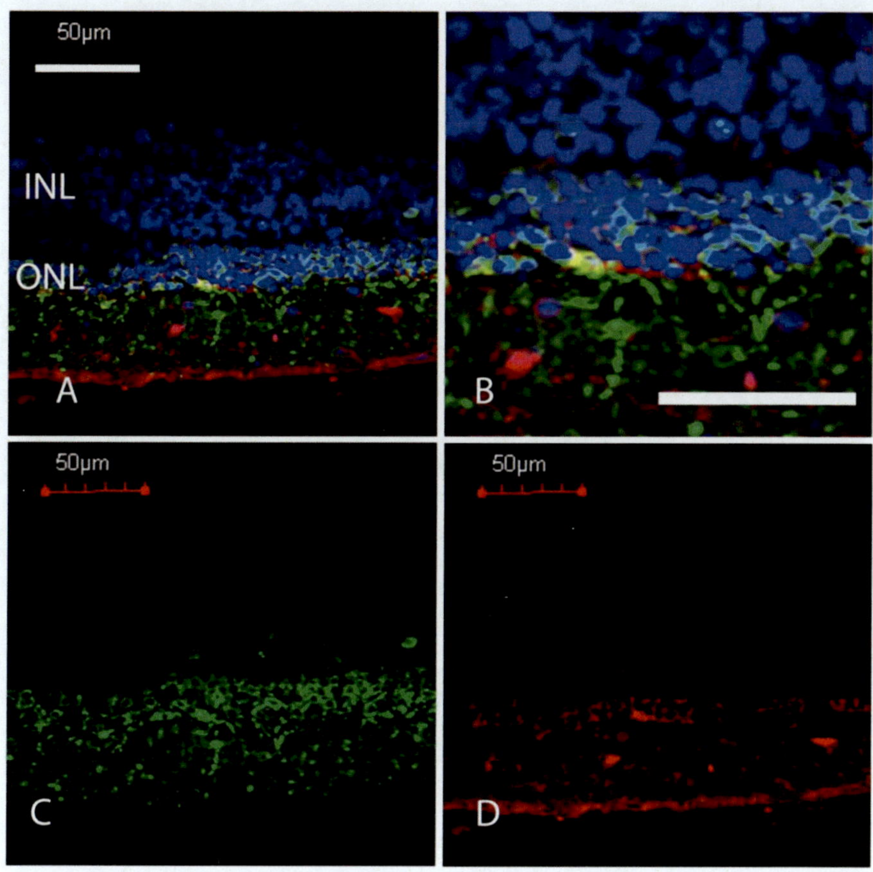

Figure 2. Thirty days after transplantation of RSCs into the subretinal space of RCS rats (60d), some Müller cells labeled with vimentin (green) in INL showed positive staining for rcoverin (red), a marker of retinal photoreceptors.A: Merged; B: zoom in; C: Vimentin staining; D : Recoverin staining. (A, C, D: scale bar = 50 µm ; B: scale bar = 25 µm). (unpublished data)

The increase of Müller cell de-differentiation may result because of the following reasons: Firstly, the transplanted stem cells may promote Müller cells to de-differentiate by an intracellular interaction such as seen in the in vitro studies. When co-clutured with retinal precursors, 60% of the cultured Müller cells de-differentiated and expressed a retinal precursor marker (Insua et al. 2008). Secondly, transplantation of retinal stem cells may bring or make the host retina generate large amounts of neurotrophic factors and transcription factors that promote the de-differentiation of Müller cells.

Studies in vitro and in vivo show that retinal stem cells secrete many kinds of cytokines and growth factors that can exert protective effects on apoptosis of retinal photoreceptors (Liljekvist-Larsson and Johansson 2005; Liljekvist-Soltic et al. 2008; Ogilvie et al. 2000). Many researchers have used cytokines or growth factors to stimulate Müller cells to re-enter the mitotic cycle and de-differentiate. These stimulating factors include EGF, Shh, Wnt, FGF and insulin (Close et al. 2006; Insua et al. 2008; Ooto et al. 2004; Osakada and Takahashi 2007; Takeda et al. 2008; Wan et al. 2008). Exogenous cell factors have also been shown to promote de-differentiation of Müller cells. Insulin, bFGF and GDNF promote cultured Müller cells to re-enter the cell cycle (Insua et al. 2008).

Ratio of de-differentiation of Müller cells

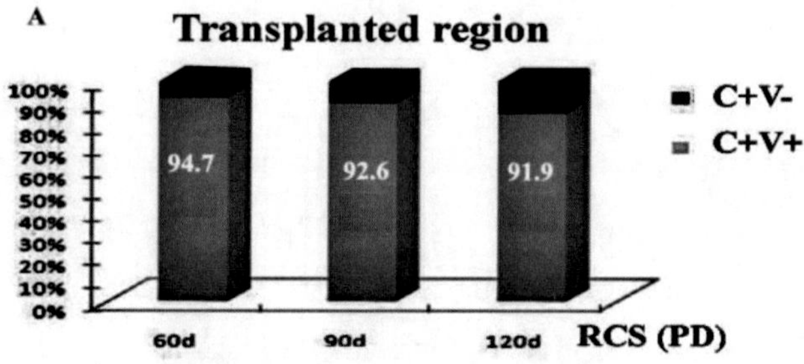

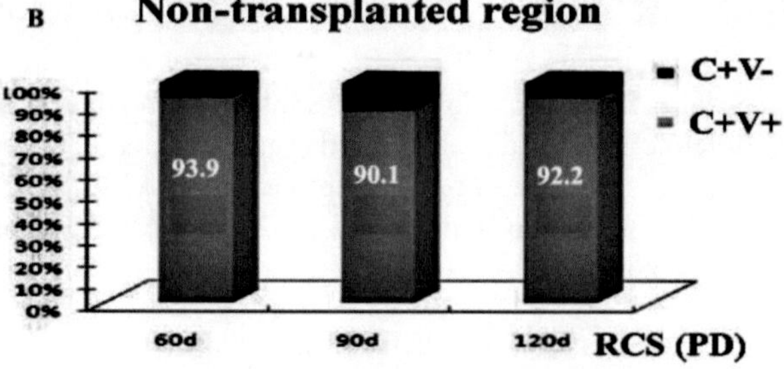

Figure 3. After RCS rats received RSCs transplants, most of Chx10 positive cells were also labeled with vimentin (C+V+). Consistently, ~10 of the population were labeled with Chx10 alone and were vimentin negative (C+V-), both in temporal retina (transplantation area) (A) and nasal retina (non-transplanted area) (B). (unpublished data).

Summary

Müller cells de-differentiate during chronic retinal degenerative diseases, and may be induced to re-differentiate into retinal neural cells after subretinal transplantation of stem cells. This maybe a major source of cell renewal in the retina, and contribute to functional retinal recovery in experimental therapy of retinal degeneration diseases.

Hypothesis

Many studies have shown that the visual function of the host in models of retinal degeneration improved after transplantation of retinal stem cells (Canola and Arsenijevic 2007; Francis et al. 2009; MacLaren et al. 2006; Seiler et al. 2008; Tomita et al. 2005). This was determined by: 1. electroretinogram (ERG) and mfERG; 2. visual evoked potentials recorded from the superior colliculus); 3. pupillary light reflexsl; and 4. ethological changes related to visual function.

From our investigation of visual function in rats and minipigs using FERG and mfERG in part III and IV, we found that transplantation of RSCs could delay progress of retinal degeneration in the RCS rat, a model of retinitis pigmentosa, and in minipigs with light-induced retinal degeneration, a model of age related macular degeneration. The visual function of whole retina was improved not only in transplanted regions but also in non transplanted regions. Why does this happen? Some studies propose that graft may set up synaptic connections with host retina and these expressed synaptophysin (Bartsch et al. 2008; MacLaren et al. 2006). But to date, there is a lack of evidence to show that these synaptophysin positive cells can connect with the host retina, and participate in transmission of a visual signal. In our study, we found that transplantation of RSCs could not only increase de-differentiation of Müller cells in the transplanted region, but also promote Müller cells de-differentiation in non transplanted region. At same time, de-differentiated Müller cells can differentiate into photoreceptors. That is, after transplantation of RSCs, not only the direct interaction of graft cells and factors, but also other factors such as cytokines released by graft cells, can increase the capacity of Müller cells to de-differentiation in the host retina. Müller cell differentiation to photoreceptors can potentially compensate for the loss of photoreceptors such as happens in retinal degeneration, thus, the visual function of host retina is improved. Based on previous work, we hypothesize that the de-differentiation of Müller cells is a common key event and a target for treatment in different retinal degeneration diseases. The subsequent re-differentiation of Müller cells into retinal neural cells after RSC subretinal transplantation will contribute a major source of renewing cells, resulting in functional retinal recovery during degenerative diseases.

Contributors

Li-Feng Chen, Shi-Ying Li, Xiao-Yong Huang, Tong-Tao Zhao, Zhong-Shan Chen, Shao-Jun Chen, Dong-Ling Liu, Chun-Yu Tian.

Acknowledgments

This work was supported by the National High Technology Research and Development Program of China (863 Program) (No. 2007AA04Z324) and the National Key Basic Scientific Research Project (973 Project) of China (2007CB512203). The authors thank Dr. Thomas FitzGibbon for his valuable comments on the research and earlier versions of the manuscript.

References

Ader, M., Meng, J., Schachner, M. & Bartsch, U. (2000). Formation of myelin after transplantation of neural precursor cells into the retina of young postnatal mice. *Glia.*, 30, 301-310

Adler, R. & Hatlee, M. (1989). Plasticity and differentiation of embryonic retinal cells after terminal mitosis. *Science.*, 243, 391-393

Ahmad, I. (2001). Stem cells: new opportunities to treat eye diseases. Invest Ophthalmol Vis Sci 42(12), 2743-8.

Ahmad, I., Das, A. V., James, J., Bhattacharya, S. & Zhao, X. (2004). Neural stem cells in the mammalian eye: types and regulation. *Semin Cell Dev Biol* 15, 53-62

Ahmad, I., Tang, L. & Pham, H. (2000). Identification of neural progenitors in the adult mammalian eye. *Biochem Biophys Res Commun.*, 270(2), 517-21.

Aramant, R. B. & Seiler, M. J. (2002). Transplanted sheets of human retina and retinal pigment epithelium develop normally in nude rats. *Exp Eye Res.*, 75: 115-125.

Arai, S., Thomas, B. B., Seiler, M. J., et al. (2004). Restoration of visual responses following transplantation of intact retinal sheets in rd mice. *Exp Eye Res.*, 79, 331-341.

Asami, M., Sun, G., Yamaguchi, M. & Kosaka, M. (2007). Multipotent cells from mammalian iris pigment epithelium. *Dev Biol.*, 304(1), 433-46.

Azadi, S., L. E. Johnson, et al. (2007). CNTF+BDNF treatment and neuroprotective pathways in the rd1 mouse retina. *Brain Res.*, 1129(1), 116-29.

Bartsch, U., Oriyakhel, W., et al. (2008). Retinal cells integrate into the outer nuclear layer and differentiate into mature photoreceptors after subretinal transplantation into adult mice. *Exp Eye Res.*, 86(4), 691-700.

Bendall, S. C., Stewart, M. H., Menendez, P., et al. (2007) IGF and FGF cooperatively establish the regulatory stem cell niche of pluripotent human cells in vitro. *Nature.*, 448: 1015-1021.

Berardi, N., Pizzorusso, T. & Maffei, L. (2004). Extracellular matrix and visual cortical plasticity: freeing the synapse. *Neuron.*, 44(6), 905-8.

Bernardos, R. L., Barthel, L. K., Meyers, J. R. & Raymond, P. A. (2007). Late-stage neuronal progenitors in the retina are radial Muller glia that function as retinal stem cells. *J Neurosci.*, 27(26), 7028-40.

Bhattacharya, S., Jackson, J. D., Das, A. V., Thoreson, W. B., Kuszynski, C., James, J., Joshi, S. & Ahmad, I. (2003). Direct identification and enrichment of retinal stem cells/progenitors by Hoechst dye efflux assay. Invest Ophthalmol Vis Sci 44(6), 2764-73.

Bochkov, N. P., Voronina, E. S., Kosyakova, N. V., Liehr, T., Rzhaninova, A. A., Katosova, L. D., Platonova, V. I. & Gol'dshtein, D. V. (2007). Chromosome variability of human multipotent mesenchymal stromal cells. *Bull Exp Biol Med.*, 143, 122-126

Canola, K., Angenieux, B., Tekaya, M., Quiambao, A., Naash, M. I., Munier, F. L., Schorderet, D. F. & Arsenijevic, Y. (2007). Retinal stem cells transplanted into models of late stages of retinitis pigmentosa preferentially adopt a glial or a retinal ganglion cell fate. *Invest Ophthalmol Vis Sci.*, 48, 446-454

Canola, K. & Arsenijevic, Y. (2007). Generation of cells committed towards the photoreceptor fate for retinal transplantation. *Neuroreport.*, 18(9), 851-5.

Cellerino, A., Bahr, M. & Isenmann, S. (2000). Apoptosis in the developing visual system. *Cell Tissue Res.*, 301(1), 53-69.

Cepko, C. L., Austin, C. P., Yang, X., Alexiades, M. & Ezzeddine, D. (1996). Cell fate determination in the vertebrate retina. *Proc Natl Acad Sci USA* 93, 589-595

Chacko, D. M., Rogers, J.A., Turner, J. E. & Ahmad, I. (2000). Survival and differentiation of cultured retinal progenitors transplanted in the subretinal space of the rat. *Biochem Biophys Res Commun*, 268, 842-846

Chandler, M. J., Smith, P. J., Samuelson, D. A., et al. (1999) Photoreceptor density of the domestic pig retina. *Vet Ophthalmol.*, 2: 179-184.

Chen, L., Yin, Z., Zeng, Y., al. e. (2007). Cryopreservation does not affect proliferation and differentiation of rats retinal stem cells. *Chinese Journal of Ocular Fundus Diseases.*, 23, 94-97.

Chen, S. J., Yin, Z. Q., Li, S. Y., et al. (2005) Comparison of microablation of choroidal tissue by LASIK and PTK Mode for neuroretina-RPE cograft sheets. *Chin J Laser Med Surg*, 14, 341-345.

Chen-xing, Z., Zheng-qin, Y., Hong-xia, X., Shi-jun, W. & Jun-ping, Y. (2005). Study on morphological characteristics in the development of the retinal ganglion cells of RCS rats. *Acta Academiae Medicinae Militaris Tertiae.*, 27(8), 749-752.

Chen, Z. S., Yin, Z. Q., Chen, S. & Wang, S. J. (2005). Electrophysiological changes of retinal ganglion cells in Royal College of Surgeons rats during retinal degeneration. *Neuroreport.*, 16(9), 971-5.

Close, J. L., Liu, J., Gumuscu, B. & Reh, T. A. (2006). Epidermal growth factor receptor expression regulates proliferation in the postnatal rat retina. *Glia.*, 54(2), 94-104.

Coles, B. L., Angenieux, B., Inoue, T., Del Rio Tsonis, K., Spence, J. R., McInnes, R. R., Arsenijevic, Y. & van der Kooy, D. (2004). Facile isolation and the characterization of human retinal stem cells. *Proc Natl Acad Sci USA.*, 101, 15772-15777

Congdon, N., O'Colmain, B., Klaver, C. C., et al. (2004) Causes and prevalence of visual impairment among adults in the United States. *Arch Ophthalmol.*, 122: 477-485.

Cui, Y. Y., Xie, H., Qi, K. B., He, Y. M. & Wang, J. F. (2004). Effects of Pinus massoniana bark extract on cell proliferation and apoptosis of human hepatoma BEL-7402 cells. *World J Gastroenterol.*, 11, 5277-5282

Das, A. V., Edakkot, S., Thoreson, W. B., James, J., Bhattacharya, S. & Ahmad, I. (2005). Membrane properties of retinal stem cells/progenitors. *Prog Retin Eye Res.*, 24(6), 663-81.

Das, A. V., James, J., Rahnenfuhrer, J., Thoreson, W. B., Bhattacharya, S., Zhao, X. & Ahmad, I. (2005a). Retinal properties and potential of the adult mammalian ciliary epithelium stem cells. *Vision Res.*, 45, 1653-1666

Di Polo, A., Cheng, L., Bray, G. M., Aguayo, A. J. (2000). Colocalization of TrkB and brain-derived neurotrophic factor proteins in green-red-sensitive cone outer segments. *Invest Ophthalmol Vis Sci.*, 41(12), 4014-21.

Djojosubroto, M. W. & Arsenijevic, Y. (2008). Retinal stem cells: promising candidates for retina transplantation. *Cell Tissue Res.*, 331(1), 347-57.

Dureau, P., Jeanny, J. C., Clerc, B. (1996). Long term light-induced retinal degeneration in the miniature pig. *Mol Vis.*, 21; 2: 7.

Eisenfeld, A. J., Bunt-Milam, A. H. & Saari, J. C. (1985). Immunocytochemical localization of interphotoreceptor retinoid-binding protein in developing normal and RCS rat retinas. *Invest Ophthalmol Vis Sci.*, 26(5), 775-8.

Engelhardt, M., Bogdahn, U. & Aigner, L. (2005). Adult retinal pigment epithelium cells express neural progenitor properties and the neuronal precursor protein doublecortin. *Brain Res.*, 1040, 98-111

Fausett, B. V., Gumerson, J. D. & Goldman, D. (2008). The proneural basic helix-loop-helix gene ascl1a is required for retina regeneration. *J Neurosci.*, 28(5), 1109-17.

Fimbel, S. M., Montgomery, J. E., Burket, C. T. & Hyde, D. R. (2007). Regeneration of inner retinal neurons after intravitreal injection of ouabain in zebrafish. *J Neurosci.*, 27(7), 1712-24.

Fischer, A. J., Reh & T. A. (2001). Muller glia are a potential source of neural regeneration in the postnatal chicken retina. *Nat Neurosci.*, 4(3), 247-52.

Florian, C., Langmann, T., Weber, B. H. & Morsczeck, C. (2008). Murine Muller cells are progenitor cells for neuronal cells and fibrous tissue cells. *Biochem Biophys Res Commun.*, 374(2), 187-91.

Francis, P. J., Wang, S., Zhang, Y., Brown, A., Hwang, T., McFarland, T. J., Jeffrey, B. G., Lu, B., Wright, L., Appukuttan, B. & others. (2009). Subretinal Transplantation of Forebrain Progenitor Cells in Non-human Primates: Survival and Intact Retinal Function. Invest Ophthalmol Vis Sci.

Friedlander, M. (2007). Fibrosis and diseases of the eye. *J Clin Invest* 117(3), 576-86.

Fujieda, H. & Sasaki, H. (2008). Expression of brain-derived neurotrophic factor in cholinergic and dopaminergic amacrine cells in the rat retina and the effects of constant light rearing. *Exp Eye Res.*, 86(2), 335-43.

Gauthier, R., Joly, S. et al. (2005). Brain-derived neurotrophic factor gene delivery to muller glia preserves structure and function of light-damaged photoreceptors. *Invest Ophthalmol Vis sci.*, 46(9), 3383-92.

Grishanin, R. N., H. Yang, et al. (2008). Retinal TrkB receptors regulate neural development in the inner, but not outer, retina. *Mol Cell Neurosci.*, 38(3), 431-43.

Hales, T. G., Tyndale, R. F. (1994). Few cell lines with GABAA mRNAs have functional receptors. *J Neurosci.*, 14(9), 5429-36.

Hanisch, U. K. & Kettenmann, H. (2007). Microglia: active sensor and versatile effector cells in the normal and pathologic brain. *Nat Neurosci.*, 10(11), 1387-94.

Haruta, M., Kosaka, M., Kanegae, Y., Saito, I., Inoue, T., Kageyama, R., Nishida, A., Honda, Y. & Takahashi, M. (2001). Induction of photoreceptor-specific phenotypes in adult mammalian iris tissue. *Nat Neurosci.*, 4(12), 1163-4.

Hegde, G. V., James, J., Das, A. V., Zhao, X., Bhattacharya, S., Ahmad, I. (2007). Characterization of early retinal progenitor microenviroment: Presence of activities selective for the differentiation of retinal ganglion cells and maintenance of progenitors. *Exp Eye Res.*, 84, 577-590.

Hims, M. M., Diager, S. P., Inglehearn, C. F. (2003). Retinitis pigmentosa: genes, proteins and prospects. *Dev Ophthalmol.*, 37, 109-25

Humayun, M. S., Prince, M., de Juan, E, Jr., Barron, Y., Moskowitz, M., Klock, I. B. & Milam, A. H. (1999). Morphometric analysis of the extramacular retina from postmortem eyes with retinitis pigmentosa. *Invest Ophthalmol Vis Sci.*, 40(1), 143-8.

Hojo, M., Abe, T., Sugano, E., Yoshioka, Y., Saigo, Y., Tomita, H., Wakusawa, R. & Tamai, M. (2004). Photoreceptor protection by iris pigment epithelial transplantation transduced with AAV-mediated brain-derived neurotrophic factor gene. *Invest Ophthalmol Vis Sci.*, 45, 3721-3726

Hood, D. C., Holopigian, K., Greenstein, V., et al. (1998). Assessment of local retinal function in patients with retinitis pigmentosa using the multi-focal ERG technique. *Vision Res.*, 38, 163-179.

Humayun, M. S., Prince, M., de Juan, E., Jr., Barron, Y., Moskowitz, M., Klock, I. B., Milam, A. H. (1999). Morphometric analysis of the extramacular retina from postmortem eyes with retinitis pigmentosa. *Invest Ophthalmol Vis Sci.*, 40(1), 143-8.

Ikeda, K., Tanihara, H. et al. (2003). Brain-dervied neurotrophic factor shows a protective effect and improves recovery of the ERG b-wave response in light-damage. *J Neurochem.*, 87(2), 290-6.

Inman., D. M. & Horner., P. J. (2007). Reactive nonproliferative gliosis predominates in a chronic mouse model of glaucoma. *Glia.*, 55(9), 942-53.

Inoue, Y., Iriyama, A., Ueno, S., et al. (2007). Subretinal transplantation of bone marrow mesenchymal stem cells delays retinal degeneration in the RCS rat model of retinal degeneration. *Exp Eye Res.*, 85, 234-241.

Insua, M. F., Simon, M. V., Garelli, A., de Los Santos, B., Rotstein, N. P. & Politi, L. E. (2008). Trophic factors and neuronal interactions regulate the cell cycle and Pax6 expression in Muller stem cells. *J Neurosci Res.*, 86(7), 1459-71.

James, J., Das, A. V., Bhattacharya, S., Chacko, D. M., Zhao, X. & Ahmad, I. (2003). In vitro generation of early-born neurons from late retinal progenitors. *J Neurosci.*, 23, 8193-8203

James, J., Das, A. V., Rahnenfuhrer, J. & Ahmad, I. (2004). Cellular and molecular characterization of early and late retinal stem cells/progenitors: differential regulation of proliferation and context dependent role of Notch signaling. *J Neurobiol.*, 61, 359-376

Jensen, R. J. & Rizzo, J. F. (2006). Thresholds for activation of rabbit retinal ganglion cells with a subretinal electrode. *Exp Eye Res.*, 83, 367-373.

Karl, M. O., Hayes, S., Nelson, B. R., Tan, K., Buckingham, B. & Reh, T. A. (2008). Stimulation of neural regeneration in the mouse retina. *Proc Natl Acad Sci U S A.*

Klassen, H. J., Ng, T. F., Kurimoto, Y., Kirov, I., Shatos, M., Coffey, P. & Young, M. J. (2004). Multipotent retinal progenitors express developmental markers, differentiate into retinal neurons, and preserve light-mediated behavior. *Invest Ophthalmol Vis Sci.*, 45(11), 4167-73.

Klassen, H., Sakaguchi, D. S. & Young, M. J. (2004b). Stem cells and retinal repair. *Prog Retin Eye Res.*, 23, 149-181

Klassen, H., Ziaeian, B., Kirov, II., Young, M. J. & Schwartz, P. H. (2004a). Isolation of retinal progenitor cells from post-mortem human tissue and comparison with autologous brain progenitors. *J Neurosci Res.*, 77, 334-343

Kohno, H., Sakai, T. & Kitahara, K. (2006). Induction of nestin, Ki-67, and cyclin D1 expression in Muller cells after laser injury in adult rat retina. *Graefes Arch Clin Exp Ophthalmol.*, 244(1), 90-5.

Kohyama, J., Abe, H., Shimazaki, T., Koizumi., A., Nakashima, K., Gojo, S., Taga, T., Okano, H., Hata, J. & Umezawa, A. (2001). Brain from bone: efficient "meta-differentiation" of marrow stroma-derived mature osteoblasts to neurons with Noggin or a demethylating agent. *Differentiation.*, 68(4-5), 235-44.

Kohyama, J., Abe, H., Shimazaki, T., Koizumi, A., Nakashima, K., Gojo, S., Taga, T., Okano, H., Hata, J. & Umezawa, A. (2001). Brain from bone: efficient "meta-differentiation" of marrow stroma-derived mature osteoblasts to neurons with Noggin or a demethylating agent. Differentiation., 68(4-5), 235-44.

Kobayashi, N., Rivas-Carrillo, J. D., Soto-Gutierrez, A., Fukazawa, T., Chen, Y., Navarro-Alvarez, N. & Tanaka, N. (2005). Gene delivery to embryonic stem cells. *Birth Defects Res C Embryo Today.*, 75, 10-18

Lakshmipathy, U., Pelacho, B., Sudo, K., Linehan, J. L., Coucouvanis, E., Kaufman, D. S. & Verfaillie, C. M. (2004). Efficient transfection of embryonic and adult stem cells. *Stem Cells.*, 22, 531-543

Landi, S., Cenni, M. C., et al. (2007). Environmental enrichment effects on development of retinal ganglion cell dendritic stratification require retinal BDNF. *PLoS ONE.*, 2(4), e346.

Landi, S., Sale, A., et al. (2007). Retinal functional development is sensitive to environmental enrichment: a role for BDNF. *FASEB J.*, 21(1), 130-9.

Layer, P. G., Robitzki, A., Rothermel, A. & Willbold, E. (2002). Of layers and spheres: the reaggregate approach in tissue engineering. *Trends Neurosci,.* 25, 131-134

Levine, E. M. & Green, E. S. (2004). Cell-intrinsic regulators of proliferation in vertebrate retinal progenitors. *Semin Cell Dev Biol.*, 15, 63-74

Li-Feng Chen, Zheng Qin Yin, Shan Chen & Chen, Z. S. (2008). Cultured stem cells from embryonic rat retina differentiate and produce action potentials in vitro. *Invest Ophthalmol Vis Sci*, 49, 5144-5150.

Liljekvist-Larsson, I. & Johansson, K. (2005). Retinal neurospheres prepared as tissue for transplantation. Brain Res Dev Brain Res 160(2):194-202.

Liljekvist-Soltic, I., Olofsson, J. & Johansson, K. (2008). Progenitor cell-derived factors enhance photoreceptor survival in rat retinal explants. *Brain Res.*, 1227, 226-33.

Lillien, L. (1995). Changes in retinal cell fate induced by overexpression of EGF receptor. *Nature.*, 377, 158–162

Liu, I. S., Chen, J. D., Ploder, L., Vidgen, D., van der Kooy, D., Kalnins, V. I. & McInnes, R. R. (1994). Developmental expression of a novel murine homeobox gene (Chx10): evidence for roles in determination of the neuroretina and inner nuclear layer. *Neuron.*, 13(2), 377-93.

Livesey, F. J., Young, T. L. & Cepko, C. L. (2004). An analysis of the gene expression program of mammalian neural progenitor cells. *Proc Natl Acad Sci USA.*, 101, 1374-1379

Liu, X., Grishanin, R. N. et al. (2007). Brain-derived neurotrophic factor and TrkB modulate visual experience-dependent refinement of neuronal pathways in retina. *J Neurosci.*, 27(27), 7256-67.

Loeliger, M. M., Briscoe, T. et al. (2008). BDNF increases survival of retinal dopaminergic neurons after prenatal compromise. *Invest Ophthalmol Vis Sci.*, 49(3), 1282-9.

Lu, L., Chen, X., Zhang, C. W., Yang, W. L., Wu, Y. J., Sun, L., Bai, L. M., Gu, X. S., Ahmed, S., Dawe, G. S. & others. (2008). Morphological and functional characterization of predifferentiation of myelinating glia-like cells from human bone marrow stromal cells through activation of F3/Notch signaling in mouse retina. *Stem Cells.*, 26(2), 580-90.

Maclaren, R. E. & Pearson, R. A. (2007). Stem cell therapy and the retina. *Eye.*, 21, 1352-1359.

MacLaren, R. E., Pearson, R. A., MacNeil, A., Douglas, R. H., Salt, T. E., Akimoto, M., Swaroop, A., Sowden, J. C. & Ali, R. R. (2006). Retinal repair by transplantation of photoreceptor precursors. *Nature.*, 444(7116), 203-7.

Maguire, A. M., Simonelli, F., Pierce, E. A., et al. (2008). Safety and efficacy of gene transfer for Leber's congenital amaurosis. *N Engl J Med,.* 358, 2240-2248.

Marler, K. J., E. Becker-Barroso, et al. (2008). A TrkB/EphrinA interaction controls retinal axon branching and synaptogenesis. *J Neurosci.*, 28(48), 12700-12.

Marmor, M. F., Hood, D. C., Keating, D., Kondo, M., Seeliger, M. W. & Miyake, Y. (2003). Guidelines for basic multifocal electroretinography (mfERG). *Doc Ophthalmol.*, 106, 105-115.

Mizumoto, H., Mizumoto, K., Shatos, M. A., Klassen, H. & Young, M.J. (2003). Retinal transplantation of neural progenitor cells derived from the brain of GFP transgenic mice. *Vision Res.*, 43, 1699-1708

Monnin, J., Morand-Villeneuve, N., Michel, G., Hicks, D. & Versaux-Botteri, C. (2007). Production of neurospheres from mammalian Muller cells in culture. *Neurosci Lett.*, 421(1), 22-6.

Nickerson, P. E., Da Silva, N., Myers, T., Stevens, K. & Clarke, D. B. (2008). Neural progenitor potential in cultured Muller glia: effects of passaging and exogenous growth factor exposure. *Brain Res.*, 1230, 1-12.

O'Brien, B. J., Isayama, T., Richardson, R. & Berson, D. M. (2002). Intrinsic physiological properties of cat retinal ganglion cells. *J Physiol.*, 538(Pt 3), 787-802.

Ogilvie, J. M., Speck, J. D. & Lett, J. M. (2000). Growth factors in combination, but not individually, rescue rd mouse photoreceptors in organ culture. *Exp Neurol.*, 161(2), 676-85.

Ooto, S., Akagi, T., Kageyama, R., Akita, J., Mandai, M., Honda, Y. & Takahashi, M. (2004). Potential for neural regeneration after neurotoxic injury in the adult mammalian retina. *Proc Natl Acad Sci U S A.*, 101(37), 13654-9.

Osakada, F. & Takahashi, M. 2007. [Stem cell therapy for the central nervous system]. *Tanpakushitsu Kakusan Koso.*, 52(5), 470-7.

Paskowitz, D. M., K. M. Donohue-Rolfe, et al. (2007). Neurotrophic factors minimize the retinal toxicity of verteporfin photodynamic therapy. *Invest Ophthalmol Vis Sci.*, 48(1), 430-7.

Pellegrini, G., De Luca, M. & Arsenijevic, Y. (2007). Towards therapeutic application of ocular stem cells. *Semin Cell Dev Biol.*, 18(6), 805-18.

Perron, M. & Harris, W. A. (2000). Retinal stem cells in vertebrates. *Bioessays* 22(8), 685-8.

Perry, V. H. & Walker, M. (1980). Morphology of cells in the ganglion cell layer during development of the rat retina. *Proc R Soc Lond B Biol Sci* 208(1173), 433-45.

Pinnock, S. B. & Herbert, J. (2008). Brain-derived neurotropic factor and neurogenesis in the adult rat dentate gyrus: interactions with corticosterone. *Eur J Neurosci.*, 27(10), 2493-500.

Qian Jian, Haiwei Xu, Hanping Xie, Yin, Z. (2009) (in press). Activation of retinal stem cells in the proliferating marginal region of RCS rats during development of retinitis pigmentosa. *Neuroscience letter.*

Qiu, G., Seiler, M. J., Mui, C., Arai, S., Aramant, R. B., de Juan Jr, E., Sadda, S. (2005). Photoreceptor differentiation and integration of retinal progenitor cells transplanted into transgenic rats. *Exp Eye Res.*, 80, 515-525

Qiu, G., Seiler, M. J., Thomas, B. B., Wu, K., Radosevich, M., Sadda, S. (2007). Revisiting nestin expression in retinal progenitor cells in vitro and after transplantation in vivo. *Exp Eye Res.*, 84, 1047-1059

Radtke, N. D., Aramant, R. B., Petry, H. M., Green, P. T., Pidwell, D. J., Seiler, M. J. Vision improvement in retinal degeneration patients by implantation of retina together with retinal pigment epithelium. *Am J Ophthalmol.*, 2008; 146, 172-182.

Raymond, P. A., Barthel, L. K., Bernardos, R. L., et al. (2006). Molecular characterization of retinal stem cells and their niches in adult zebrafish. *BMC Devel Biol.*, 6: 36.

Reh, T. A. (2002). Neural stem cells: form and function. Nat Neurosci 5(5):392-4.

Reh, T. A., Fischer, A. J. (2001). Stem cells in the vertebrate retina. *Brain Behav Evol.*, 58, 296-305

Reh, T. A. & Kljavin, I. J. (1989). Age of differentiation determines rat retinal germinal cell phenotype: induction of differentiation by dissociation. *J Neurosci.*, 9, 4179–4189

Rickman, D. W. & Brecha, N. C. (1995). Expression of the proto-oncogene, trk, receptors in the developing rat retina. *Vis Neurosci.*, 12(2), 215-22.

Robinson, D. W. & Wang, G. Y. (1998). Development of intrinsic membrane properties in mammalian retinal ganglion cells. *Semin Cell Dev Biol.*, 9(3), 301-10.

Rohrer, B., Korenbrot, J. I., LaVail, M. M., Reichardt, L. F. & Xu, B. (1999). Role of neurotrophin receptor TrkB in the maturation of rod photoreceptors and establishment of synaptic transmission to the inner retina. *J Neurosci.*, 19(20), 8919-30.

Salasznyka, R. M., Kleesa, R. F., Williamsa, W. A., Boskeyb, A. & Plopper, G. E. (2007). Focal adhesion kinase signaling pathways regulate the osteogenic differentiation of human mesenchymal stem cells. *Exp Cell Res.*, 313, 22–37

Sakaguchi, D. S., Van Hoffelen, S. J., Theusch, E., et al. (2004) Transplantation of neural progenitor cells into the developing retina of the Brazilian opossum: an in vivo system for studying stem/progenitor cell plasticity. *Dev Neurosci.*, 26, 336-345.

Schmid, S. & Guenther, E. (1998). Alterations in channel density and kinetic properties of the sodium current in retinal ganglion cells of the rat during in vivo differentiation. *Neuroscience.*, 85(1), 249-58.

Schwartz, P. H., Bryant, P. J., Fuja, T. J., Su, H., O'Dowd, D. K. & Klassen, H. (2003). Isolation and characterization of neural progenitor cells from post-mortem human cortex. *J Neurosci Res.*, 74, 838–851

Schwartz, P. H., Nethercott, H., Kirov, I. I., Ziaeian, B., Young, M. J., Klassen, H. (2005). Expression of neurodevelopmental markers by cultured porcine neural precursor cells. *Stem Cells.*, 23, 1286-1294

Seiler, M. J., Thomas, B. B., Chen, Z., Arai, S., Chadalavada, S., Mahoney, M. J., Sadda, S. R., Aramant & R. B. (2008). BDNF-treated retinal progenitor sheets transplanted to degenerate rats: improved restoration of visual function. *Exp Eye Res.*, 86(1), 92-104.

Shatz, C. J. (1996). Emergence of order in visual system development. *Proc Natl Acad Sci U S A.*, 93(2), 602-8.

Sieving, P. A., Caruso, R. C., Tao, W., et al. (2006). Ciliary neurotrophic factor (CNTF) for human retinal degeneration: phase I trial of CNTF delivered by encapsulated cell intraocular implants. *Proc Natl Acad Sci USA.*, 103, 3896-3901.

Skaliora, I., Robinson, D. W., Scobey, R. P. & Chalupa, L. M. (1995). Properties of K+ conductances in cat retinal ganglion cells during the period of activity-mediated refinements in retinofugal pathways. *Eur J Neurosci.*, 7(7), 1558-68.

Song, H. J., Stevens, C. F. & Gage, F. H. (2002). Neural stem cells from adult hippocampus develop essential properties of functional CNS neurons. *Nat Neurosci.*, 5(5), 438-45.

Sucher, N. J., Brose, N., Deitcher, D. L., Awobuluyi, M., Gasic, G. P., Bading, H., Cepko, C. L., Greenberg, M. E., Jahn, R., Heinemann, S. F. & others. (1993). Expression of endogenous NMDAR1 transcripts without receptor protein suggests post-transcriptional control in PC12 cells. *J Biol Chem.*, 268(30), 22299-304.

Sun, W., Buzanska, L., Domanska-Janik, K., Salvi, R. J., Stachowiak, M. K. (2005). Voltage-sensitive and ligand-gated channels in differentiating neural stem-like cells derived from the nonhematopoietic fraction of human umbilical cord blood. *Stem Cells.*, 23(7), 931-45.

Takeda, M., Takamiya, A., Jiao, J. W., Cho, K. S., Trevino, S. G., Matsuda, T., Chen, D. F. (2008). alpha-Aminoadipate induces progenitor cell properties of Muller glia in adult mice. *Invest Ophthalmol Vis Sci.*, 49(3), 1142-50.

Thummel, R., Kassen, S. C., Enright, J. M., Nelson, C. M., Montgomery, J. E. & Hyde, D. R. (2008a). Characterization of Muller glia and neuronal progenitors during adult zebrafish retinal regeneration. *Exp Eye Res.*, 87(5), 433-44.

Thummel, R., Kassen, S. C., Montgomery, J. E., Enright, J. M. & Hyde, D. R. (2008b). Inhibition of Muller glial cell division blocks regeneration of the light-damaged zebrafish retina. *Dev Neurobiol.*, 68(3), 392-408.

Tomita, M., Lavik, E., Klassen, H., Zahir, T., Langer, R. & Young, M. J. (2005). Biodegradable polymer composite grafts promote the survival and differentiation of retinal progenitor cells. *Stem Cells*, 23(10), 1579-88.

Tropepe, V., Coles, B. L., Chiasson, B. J., Horsford, D. J., Elia, A. J., McInnes, R. R. & van der Kooy, D. (2000). Retinal stem cells in the adult mammalian eye. *Science.*, 287, 2032-2036

Villegas-Perez, M. P., Lawrence, J. M., Vidal-Sanz, M., Lavail, M. M., Lund, R. D. (1998). Ganglion cell loss in RCS rat retina: a result of compression of axons by contracting intraretinal vessels linked to the pigment epithelium. *J Comp Neurol.*, 392(1), 58-77.

Vissio, P. G. & Canepa, M. M. et al. (2008). Brain-derived neurotrophic factor (BDNF)-like immunoreactivity localization in the retina and brain of Cichlasoma dimerus (Teleostei, Perciformes). *Tissue Cell.*, 40(4), 261-70.

Wang, D. Y., Chan., W. M., Tam, P. O., Baum, L., Lam, D. S., Chong, K. K., Fan, B. J. & Pang, C. P. (2005). Gene mutations in retinitis pigmentosa and their clinical implications. *Clin Chim Acta.*, 351(1-2), 5-16.

Wang, F., Wang, Z. & Sun, X., et al. (2004). Safety and efficacy of dispase and plasmin in pharmacologic vitreolysis. *Invest Ophthalmol Vis Sci.*, 45: 3286-3290.

Wang, S., Girman, S., Lu, B., et al. (2008). Long-term vision rescue by human neural progenitors in a rat model of photoreceptor degeneration. *Invest Ophthalmol Vis Sc.*, 49, 3201-3206.

Wang, S., Girman, S., et al. (2008). Long-term vision rescue by human neural progenitors in a rat model of photoreceptor degeneration. *Invest Ophthalmol Vis Sci.*, 49(7), 3201-6.

Wan, J., Zheng, H., Chen, Z. L., Xiao, H. L., Shen, Z. J. & Zhou, G. M. (2008). Preferential regeneration of photoreceptor from Muller glia after retinal degeneration in adult rat. *Vision Res.*, 48(2), 223-34.

Warren, R. A. & Jones, E. G. (1997). Maturation of neuronal form and function in a mouse thalamo-cortical circuit. *J Neurosci.*, 17(1), 277-95.

Weber, A. J. & Harman, C. D. (2008). BDNF preserves the dendritic morphology of alpha and beta ganglion cells in the cat retina after optic nerve injury. *Invest Ophthalmol Vis Sci.*, 49(6), 2456-63.

Wegner, M., Stolt, C. C. (2005). From stem cells to neurons and glia: a Soxist's view of neural development. Trends Neurosci 28(11):583-8.

West, E. L., R. A. Pearson, et al. (2008). Pharmacological disruption of the outer limiting membrane leads to increased retinal integration of transplanted photoreceptor precursors. Exp Eye Res 86(4): 601-11.

Wojciechowski, A. B., Englund, U., Lundberg, C., Wictorin, K., Warfvinge, K. (2002). Subretinal transplantation of brain-derived precursor cells to young RCS rats promotes photoreceptor cell survival. *Exp Eye Res*, 75, 23-37

Wu, Z. Z. & Pan, H. L. (2004). Tetrodotoxin-sensitive and -resistant Na+ channel currents in subsets of small sensory neurons of rats. *Brain Res* 1029(2), 251-8.

Xuan, A. G., Long, D. H. et al. (2008). BDNF improves the effects of neural stem cells on the rat model of Alzheimer's disease with unilateral lesion of fimbria-fornix. *Neurosci Lett.*, 440(3), 331-5.

Yamasaki, E. N., Ramoa, A. S. (1993). Dendritic remodelling of retinal ganglion cells during development of the rat. *J Comp Neurol.*, 329(2), 277-89.

Yanagi, Y., Inoue, Y., Kawase, Y., Uchida, S., Tamaki, Y., Araie, M., Okochi, H. (2006). Properties of growth and molecular profiles of rat progenitor cells from ciliary epithelium. *Exp Eye Res*, 82, 471-478

Yang, P., Seiler, M. J., Aramant, R. B., Whittemore, S. (2002). Differential lineage restriction of ratretinal progenitor cells in vitro and in vivo. *J Neurosci Res.*, 69, 466-476

Yoshimura, N. (2001). [Retinal neuronal cell death: molecular mechanism and neuroprotection]. *Nippon Ganka Gakkai Zasshi.*, 105(12), 884-902.

Yu, D. Y., Cringle, S. J., Su, E. N., Yu, P. K. (2000). Intraretinal oxygen levels before and after photoreceptor loss in the RCS rat. *Invest Ophthalmol Vis Sci.*, 41, 3999-4006

Zahir, T., Klassen, H., Young, M. J. (2005). Effects of ciliary neurotrophic factor on differentiation of late retinal progenitor cells. *Stem Cells.*, 23, 424-432

Zahir, T., Klassen, H., Tomita, M., Young, M. J. (2006). Sorbitol causes preferential selection of Muller glial precursors from late retinal progenitor cells in vitro. *Mol Vis*, 12, 1606-1614

Zhang, Y., Arner, K. et al. (2003). Limitation of anatomical integration between subretinal transplants and the host retina. *Invest Ophthalmol Vis Sci.*, 44(1), 324-31.

Zhao, S., Thornquist, S. C., Barnstable, C. J. (1995). In vitro transdifferentiation of embryonic rat retinal pigment epithelium to neural retina. *Brain Res.*, 677, 300-310

In: Reginitis Pigmentosa: Causes, Diagnosis…   ISBN: 978-1-60876-884-4
Editors: M. Baert, et al. pp. 65-88   © 2010 Nova Science Publishers, Inc.

Retinitis Pigmentosa

Eleftherios Papathanasiou
The Cyprus Institute of Neurology & Genetics, Nicosia, Cyprus.

Abstract

Retinis Pigmentosa (RP) is a term that includes a group of progressive hereditary retinal diseases involving degeneration of rod and cone photoreceptors, predominantly the former, and is one of the leading causes of hereditary blindness in the developed world. Ganglion cells are also affected, possibly due to transsynaptic neuronal damage caused by loss of neuronal input from the degenerating photoreceptor cell layer. Clinical symptoms include nyctalopia, progressive visual field loss, and deterioration in visual acuity in adolescence. No effective therapy exists at present. It affects one in 3000-5000 individuals and can be caused by mutations in more than 40 genes. Retinitis Pigmentosa may exist either alone (nonsyndromic) or as part of a neurological or systemic disorder, such as Usher's syndrome and Infantile Refsum's disease. Typical findings on retinal examination include retinal vessel attenuation. Bone spicule formation is also noted around the intraretinal vessels (pigmentary clumping), caused by the hyperplasia and migration of retinal pigment epithelial cells into the inner layers of the neurosensory retina. The disease may be inherited as either autosomal recessive, autosomal dominant or X-linked. Autosomal dominant inheritance is the most common. Several mechanisms to explain the degeneration process have been proposed. These include misfolding of the rod visual pigment

Rhodopsin preventing its transportation to the outer segment, dysfunction of cell transport systems that are involved with photoreceptor protein localization, starvation of cones and cyclic GMP-dependent protein kinase activation. Therapies that are currently under investigation include the use of ribozymes for the targeted reduction of mutant-allele mRNA and the use of retinoids to improve protein folding.

Retinis Pigmentosa (RP) is a term that includes a group of progressive hereditary retinal diseases involving degeneration of rod and cone photoreceptors, predominantly the former, and is one of the leading causes of hereditary blindness in the developed world. It is regarded as an apoptotic phenomenon (Tuson et al., 2009), although non-apoptotic mechanisms have been suggested (Sancho-Pelluz et al., 2008). It was first described by van Trigt in 1853, and named retinitis pigmentosa by Donders in the Netherlands (Donders, 1857; Birch, 2006). Rod photoreceptor cell degeneration precedes cone photoreceptor degeneration (Mendes et al., 2005). Ganglion cells are also affected, possibly due to transynaptic neuronal damage caused by loss of neuronal input from the degenerating photoreceptor cell layer (Newman et al., 1987; Flannery et al., 1989; Janaky et al., 2008). Clinical symptoms include nyctalopia, progressive visual field loss, and deterioration in visual acuity in adolescence (Goodwin, 2008). There is progressive field constriction with relative preservation of macular function (Birch, 2006). It affects one in 3000-5000 individuals (over 1.5 million peoples worldwide) and can be caused by mutations in more than 40 genes (Chiang et al., 2006). More than 20 mutations associated with RP have been identified in the RP1 gene, all of them leading to the production of a truncated protein without 50-70% of the C-terminal of the RP1 protein (Chiang et al., 2006). Retinitis Pigmentosa may exist either alone (nonsyndromic) or as part of a neurological or systemic disorder, such as Usher's syndrome and Infantile Refsum's disease. Typical findings on retinal examination include retinal vessel attenuation. Bone spicule formation is also noted around the intraretinal vessels (pigmentary clumping), caused by the hyperplasia and migration of retinal pigment epithelial cells into the inner layers of the neurosensory retina. Clinically, foveal dysfunction in RP manifests as reduced visual acuity (Grover et al., 1996), which is thought to be due to the reduced spatial density of the foveal cones found during histological studies of the maculae of RP donor eyes (Flannery et al., 1989; Stone et al., 1992; Santos et al., 1997; Alexander et al.,

2005). Reduced visual acuity has been found to be correlated with a reduced perception of quality of life (Sugawara et al., 2009). The progression of retinitis pigmentosa is not influenced by pregnancy (Vingolo et al., 2009). The only significant result found in this study was a slight worsening of visual acuity at 5 months post partum. The authors explain that if this is truly significant, this may be because all of the patients breastfed their children and might have undergone a depletion of vitamin A and docosahexanoic acid.

Mechanisms of Inheritance

The disease may be inherited as either autosomal recessive (5-20%), autosomal dominant (15-25%), X-linked (5-15%) or sporadic (40-50%) (Bunker et al., 1984; Birch, 2006; Chiang et al., 2006). Autosomal dominant inheritance has been reported to be the most common (Goodwin, 2008) and the mildest (Shastry, 1994). Even though many mutations have been found that involve several proteins (Table 1), the mutations themselves may not be the only cause of the disease. For example, in relation to rhodopsin mutations, the vast majority of which cause the autosomal dominant type (Mendes et al., 2005), a wide variety of clinical expression can be seen even within a family with the same mutation, and their late onset, slow progression and cone degeneration suggest that other factors or genes (modifier genes) in addition to rhodopsin are responsible for the phenotypic expression of the disorder (Shastry, 1994). However, so far no modifier genes have been located (Goodwin, 2008). A list of the proteins known to be dysfunctional due to DNA mutations are shown in Table 1.

RP associated with Other Systemic Diseases

In most cases RP is seen in isolation (nonsyndromic) (Birch, 2006), but in some cases it may be a part of a genetic, metabolic, or neurologic syndrome or disorder (Bhatti, 2006). These are listed in Table 2.

Table 1. Listed below are proteins that have been found to be dysfunctional in RP patients based on DNA mutation analysis, together with their known function and what the mutated protein eventually does in the human retina.

Mutated protein	Function	Mutation Effect	References
Rhodopsin (RHO) (over 120 mutations)	Transmembrane protein that initiates visual transduction cascade when photoexcited.	Protein misfolding and mislocalisation.	Dryja et al., 1990; Farrar et al., 1990; al-Maghtheh et al., 1993; Mendes et al., 2005; Mendes and Cheetham 2008.
Peripherin (RDS)	Required for proper formation of the specialized outer segment organelle	Lack of photoreceptor outer segment formation	van Nie et al, 1978; Farjo and Naash, 2006
RP1 (over 20 mutations)	Rhodopsin transport, microtubule-associated protein	Mislocalisation of rhodopsin to inner segments and cell bodies	Chiang et al., 2006.
RP2	DNA binding protein with exonuclease activity	Unknown	Yoon et al., 2006
RP GTPase Regulator (RPGR) or RP3	Specific role in rod and cone survival intersegmental transport.	Mis-localization of opsin-containing vesicles	Hong et al., 2000; He et al., 2008; Neidhardt et al., 2008
NRL	Photoreceptor gene regulation	Altered expression of Rhodopsin	Yang-Feng and Swaroop, 1992; Rehemtulla et al., 1996.
CNGA1	Rod cGMP-gated channel	Lack of channels, or accumulation inside rod inner segment	Dryja et al., 1995.
RLBP1	Cellular retinaldehyde-binding protein	Delayed dark adaption, other functions unclear	Morimura et al., 1999; Humbert et al., 2006.

In: Reginitis Pigmentosa: Causes, Diagnosis...   ISBN: 978-1-60876-884-4
Editors: M. Baert, et al. pp. 65-88   © 2010 Nova Science Publishers, Inc.

Chapter II

Retinitis Pigmentosa

Eleftherios Papathanasiou
The Cyprus Institute of Neurology & Genetics, Nicosia, Cyprus.

Abstract

Retinis Pigmentosa (RP) is a term that includes a group of progressive hereditary retinal diseases involving degeneration of rod and cone photoreceptors, predominantly the former, and is one of the leading causes of hereditary blindness in the developed world. Ganglion cells are also affected, possibly due to transsynaptic neuronal damage caused by loss of neuronal input from the degenerating photoreceptor cell layer. Clinical symptoms include nyctalopia, progressive visual field loss, and deterioration in visual acuity in adolescence. No effective therapy exists at present. It affects one in 3000-5000 individuals and can be caused by mutations in more than 40 genes. Retinitis Pigmentosa may exist either alone (nonsyndromic) or as part of a neurological or systemic disorder, such as Usher's syndrome and Infantile Refsum's disease. Typical findings on retinal examination include retinal vessel attenuation. Bone spicule formation is also noted around the intraretinal vessels (pigmentary clumping), caused by the hyperplasia and migration of retinal pigment epithelial cells into the inner layers of the neurosensory retina. The disease may be inherited as either autosomal recessive, autosomal dominant or X-linked. Autosomal dominant inheritance is the most common. Several mechanisms to explain the degeneration process have been proposed. These include misfolding of the rod visual pigment

Rhodopsin preventing its transportation to the outer segment, dysfunction of cell transport systems that are involved with photoreceptor protein localization, starvation of cones and cyclic GMP-dependent protein kinase activation. Therapies that are currently under investigation include the use of ribozymes for the targeted reduction of mutant-allele mRNA and the use of retinoids to improve protein folding.

Retinis Pigmentosa (RP) is a term that includes a group of progressive hereditary retinal diseases involving degeneration of rod and cone photoreceptors, predominantly the former, and is one of the leading causes of hereditary blindness in the developed world. It is regarded as an apoptotic phenomenon (Tuson et al., 2009), although non-apoptotic mechanisms have been suggested (Sancho-Pelluz et al., 2008). It was first described by van Trigt in 1853, and named retinitis pigmentosa by Donders in the Netherlands (Donders, 1857; Birch, 2006). Rod photoreceptor cell degeneration precedes cone photoreceptor degeneration (Mendes et al., 2005). Ganglion cells are also affected, possibly due to transynaptic neuronal damage caused by loss of neuronal input from the degenerating photoreceptor cell layer (Newman et al., 1987; Flannery et al., 1989; Janaky et al., 2008). Clinical symptoms include nyctalopia, progressive visual field loss, and deterioration in visual acuity in adolescence (Goodwin, 2008). There is progressive field constriction with relative preservation of macular function (Birch, 2006). It affects one in 3000-5000 individuals (over 1.5 million peoples worldwide) and can be caused by mutations in more than 40 genes (Chiang et al., 2006). More than 20 mutations associated with RP have been identified in the RP1 gene, all of them leading to the production of a truncated protein without 50-70% of the C-terminal of the RP1 protein (Chiang et al., 2006). Retinitis Pigmentosa may exist either alone (nonsyndromic) or as part of a neurological or systemic disorder, such as Usher's syndrome and Infantile Refsum's disease. Typical findings on retinal examination include retinal vessel attenuation. Bone spicule formation is also noted around the intraretinal vessels (pigmentary clumping), caused by the hyperplasia and migration of retinal pigment epithelial cells into the inner layers of the neurosensory retina. Clinically, foveal dysfunction in RP manifests as reduced visual acuity (Grover et al., 1996), which is thought to be due to the reduced spatial density of the foveal cones found during histological studies of the maculae of RP donor eyes (Flannery et al., 1989; Stone et al., 1992; Santos et al., 1997; Alexander et al.,

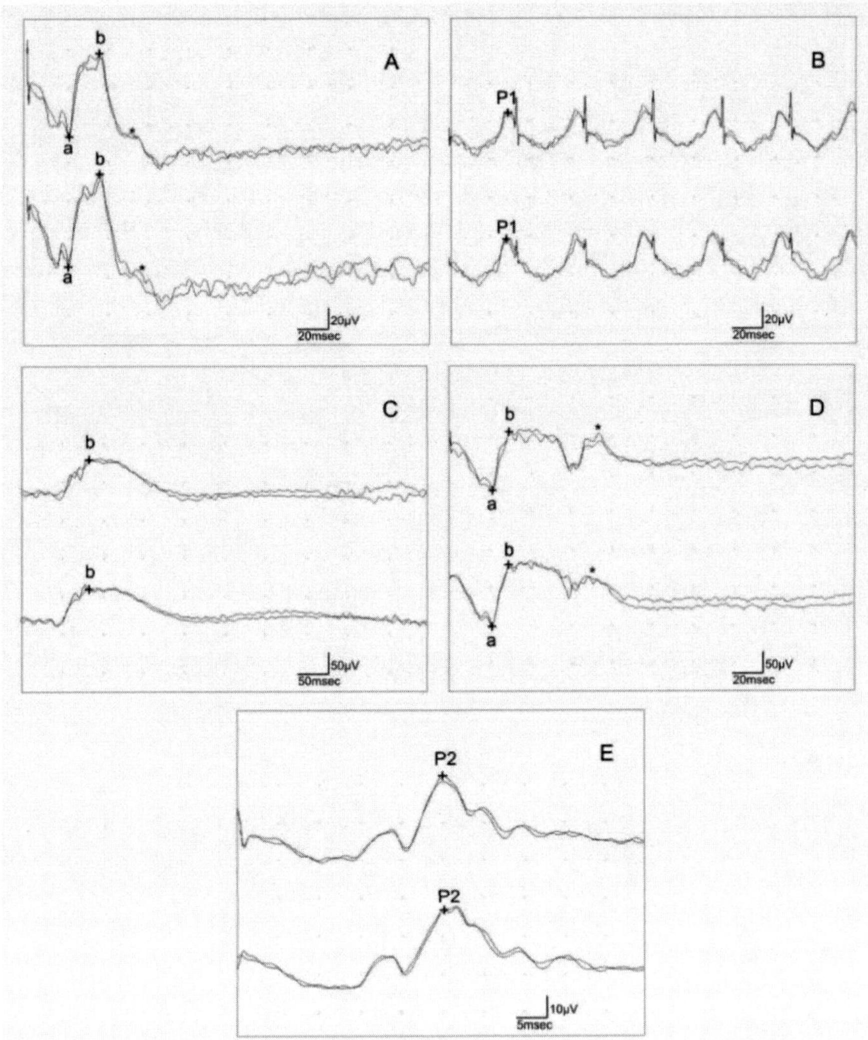

Figure 1. Standard flash cone (A), 30 Hz flicker (B), rod (C), standard combined (D) and oscillatory (E) responses in a physiologically normal volunteer. Two responses are shown superimposed for each protocol, with the top tracing in each protocol representing the response from the left eye, and the bottom tracing from that of the right eye. 3-5 stimulations were obtained and averaged for each tracing. Reproduced from Papathanasiou and Papacostas, 2008, with kind permission of Springer Science and Business Media.

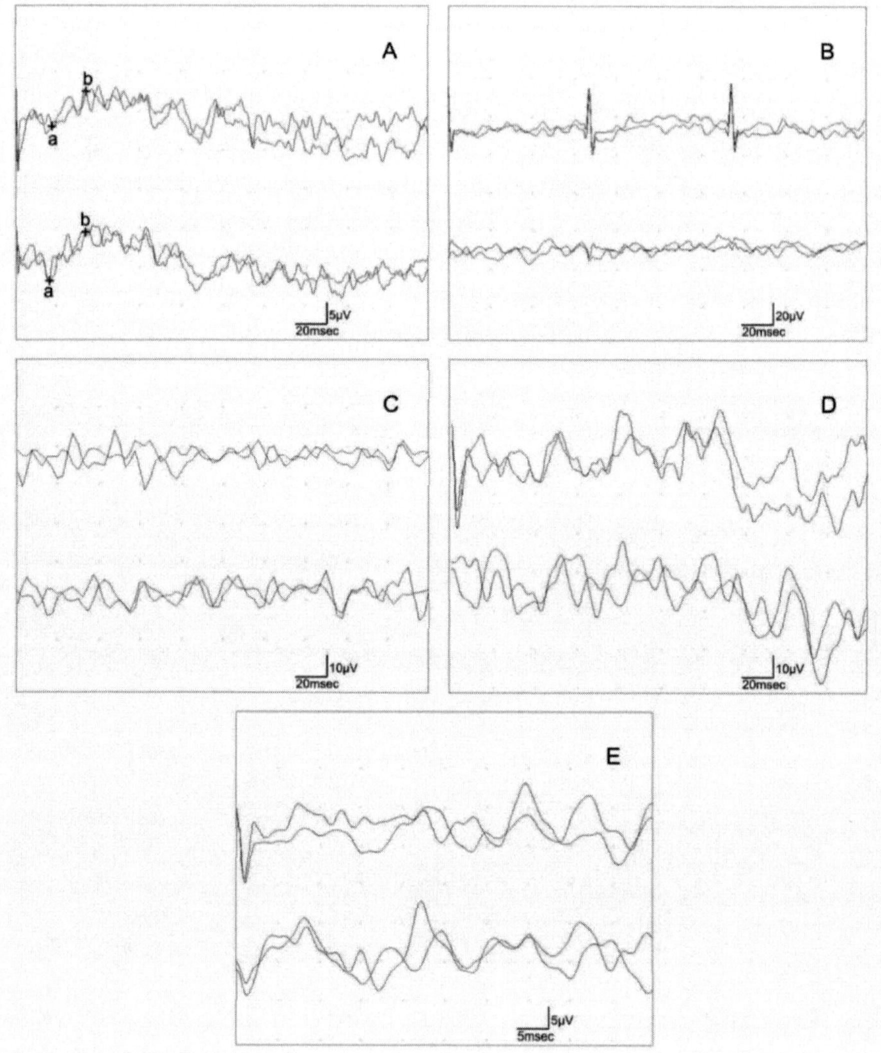

Figure 2. Responses from a patient with Retinitis Pigmentosa. The annotations are as in figure 1. The patient showed low amplitude standard flash cone and oscillatory responses, and unobtainable standard flash rod, standard combined and flicker responses. Reproduced from Papathanasiou and Papacostas, 2008, with kind permission of Springer Science and Business Media.

dependent on the type of mutation. For example, the mean annual exponential rate of decline for the 30 Hz cone FERG amplitude is faster for the USH2A mutation related to Usher syndrome type II than for the RHO and RPGR mutations (Sandberg et al., 2008). However, the rate of acuity loss due to USH2A mutations fell between the latter two. X-linked RP is more severely affected. It has been found that only 41% of patients have a recordable FERG (Paranhos et al., 1998-99). An example of a recording in a patient with RP is shown in figure 2. A unique ERG pattern may exist that may represent an intermediate stage in deterioration, with wavelets or small waves making up the ERG response in both dark and light adapted conditions (Lam et al., 1999; Aleman et al., 2009).

Pattern electroretinography (PERG)

The pattern electroretinogram (PERG) is a retinal biopotential that is evoked when a temporally modulated patterned stimulus of constant total luminance (checkerboard or grating) is viewed (Bach et al., 2006). The PERG is a very small signal, typically in the region of 0.5-8 uV depending on stimulus characteristics, and PERG is technically more demanding than the conventional ERG.

Studies have shown that the PERG is never normal in RP patients (Janaky et al., 2008). 68% of patients have been shown to yield unobtainable responses. The remaining patients revealed responses of low amplitude, with some responses showing increased P50 absolute latencies.

Multifocal electroretinography (mfERG)

Multifocal electroretinography (mfERG) is a new technique that allows analysis of local retinal function (Marmor et al., 2006). It assesses local ERG from different regions of the posterior retina. Electrical responses from the eye are recorded with a corneal electrode and produce a topographical map of ERG responses. The retina is stimulated with a computer monitor or other device that generates a pattern of elements (typically hexagons), each of which has a 50% chance of being illuminated every time the frame changes. Each element follows a fixed, predetermined sequence, while at the same time keeping the overall luminance of the monitor stable. The mfERG waveforms are a mathematical extraction of signals that correlate with the time that one portion of the stimulus screen is illuminated.

The mfERG can be abnormal in X-linked RP carriers in females, even in the presence of normal full-field ERG recordings (Vingolo et al., 2006). This is due to the fact that, according to a hypothesis proposed by Lyon, carriers of an X-linked trait would be expected to exhibit greater variability because early in embryonic development, one x-chromosome, independently in each cell of a female, becomes inactive. As a consequence the tissue of a heterozygote female becomes a mosaic of cells with some cells expressing a normal and others expressing an abnormal gene (Lyon, 1961). The full-field ERG does not allow resolution of the responses from discrete retinal areas, and small loci of retinal dysfunction may not alter the full-field ERG.The mfERG demonstrated patchy areas of retinal dysfunction in some carriers of XLRP with normal full-field ERG (amplitude and implicit time) (Vajaranant et al., 2002). One advantage of the mfERG in patients with RP is that it can be recorded in advanced cases, even if the FERG is unobtainable (Nagy et al., 2008). It allows a long-term follow-up of disease progression, and it can also be used as an objective outcome measure in upcoming treatment studies involving patients with advanced retinal diseases. One study has found greater intertrial variability in RP patients than in normal controls when using mfERG (Seiple et al., 2004), and it has therefore advised evaluating repeat studies on an individual basis.

Pattern visual evoked potentials (PVEPs)

Evoked potentials are reliable diagnostic tests that yield reproducible results in routine clinical practice (Chiappa, 1997). They provide an objective measure of function in their related sensory systems and tracts. The clinical utility of evoked potentials is based on their ability (1) to demonstrate abnormal sensory system function when the history and/or neurological examination are equivocal; (2) to reveal the presence of clinically unsuspected malfunction in a sensory system when demyelinating disease is suspected because of symptoms and/or signs in another area of the central nervous system; (3) to help define the anatomic distribution of a disease process; and (4) to monitor changes objectively over time in a patient's status.

An evoked potential is an electrical manifestation of the brain's reception of and response to an external stimulus. Seperation of the buried evoked potential waveforms from the other electrical activity is accomplished by signal averaging. Since the electrical response of the brain to the stimulus always comes at the same interval of time after the stimulus, simple computers (signal averagers) can be used to extract the desired signal (the evoked potential) from the temporally random background activity. Stimuli are given repetitively and the computer averages the new data acquired after each stimulus (random EEG plus evoked potential) with the averaged results from previous stimuli stored in its memory. The process is continued until the desired waveform becomes sufficiently clarified.

The current standard presents basic responses elicited by three commonly used stimulus conditions using a single, midline recording channel with an occipital, active electrode (Odom et al., 2004). Pattern reversal of a black and white checkerboard pattern is the preferred technique for most clinical purposes.

Although the rod system appears to be the target of the disease, the foveal cone system can also be affected (Alexander et al., 2005) and is therefore expected to affect the PVEP. The PVEP has been used to show that both the parvocellular (colour, high contrast black and white stimuli) and magnocellular (transient motion, low contrast black and white stimuli) pathways are involved (Alexander et al., 2005).

PVEPs can be recorded in all patients (Paranhos et al., 1998-1999; Janaky et al., 2008). In one study, 32% would reveal normal P100 waveform shape, low amplitude responses, with P100 absolute latency only slightly prolonged in the majority of these cases (Janaky et al., 2008). Interestingly, 30% revealed a characteristic bifid pattern that has been associated in other studies with demyelination (Rousseff et al., 2005). It was not demonstrated in this study whether the use of half-field stimulation (top field) removed one or the other peak to help in the placement of the P100 marker, which can sometimes help in removing one of the peaks that may be a contamination from the Fz reference electrode (Chiappa and Hill, 1997). The remaining 38% showed long duration waveforms of prolonged P100 absolute latency, with most of the responses of low amplitude. No association was found between the different types of recordings and the duration of RP or the extent of the visual field defect. Low amplitude responses in all RP patients at all check sizes have also been found in another study (Paranhos et al., 1998-1999).

Optical Coherence Tomography (OCT)

Optical coherence tomography (OCT) is a rapid non-contact method that allows in vivo imaging of the retina, optic nerve head and retinal nerve fibre layer (RNFL) (Sakata et al., 2009). Since its introduction in Ophthalmology approximately a decade ago, the use of this technology has disseminated into the clinical practice. OCT has proven to be a useful ancillary tool for assessing retinal diseases because of its capability to provide cross-sectional images of the retina, and also to perform quantitative analysis of retinal morphology.

The use of OCT has revealed an increase in the thickness of the retinal ganglion cell layer in some RP patients and a thicker retinal nerve fiber layer in the majority of patients (Hood et al., 2008). The effects here also depend on the type of mutation, with RPGR mutations related to autosomal dominant inheritance leading to a greater loss of foveal cones when compared with RHO mutations (Goodwin, 2008). In addition, OCT also showed early outer nuclear layer thinning with inner nuclear thickening in patients with X-linked RP with RPGR mutations. Thinning of the retinal nerve fiber layer was found to be directly correlated with the severity of the pallor of the optic disc, but not with the remaining visual field (Walia et al., 2007), refractive error or visual acuity (Oishi et al., 2009). The paradoxical thickening noted in the inner nuclear layer may be related to Müller glial activation with hypertrophy (Milam et al., 1998; Humayun et al., 1999; Aleman et al., 2008). With the use of OCT, a disease sequence for the development of RP has been proposed, consisting of initial outer nuclear layer diminution with inner nuclear layer thickening, followed by amalgamation of residual outer nuclear layer with the thickened inner nuclear layer, and ending up with progressive retinal remodelling and eventual thinning (Aleman et al., 2008). The latter thinning leads to the disappearance of normal retinal lamination and is probably due to migrating retinal pigment epithelium interspersed with neural and glial cells and neurite sprouting. OCT can reveal the presence of cystoid macular edema in a significant percentage of RP patients with no fundoscopic evidence of cystic macular lesions (Hajali and Fishman, 2008). As visual acuity has been shown to be influenced by edema in the parafovea as well as in the fovea (Sandberg et al., 2008), knowing the presence of this edema will lead to its therapeutic **removal and increase in the patient's visual acuity.** All X-linked RP carriers and affected males show abnormalities in OCT which consists of macular edema and increased RPE reflectivity, compared to no alterations in unaffected females (Vingolo et al., 2006).

Possible Causes of Retinitis Pigmentosa

Several mechanisms to explain the degeneration process have been proposed. But most of the proposed mechanisms are believed to result in apoptosis of rod photoreceptors. Apoptosis is programmed cell death as signalled by the nuclei in normally functioning human and animal cells when age or state of cell health and condition dictates. It is an active process requiring metabolic activity by the dying cell, often characterised by cleavage of the DNA into fragments that give a so called laddering pattern on gels. Cells that die by apoptosis do not usually elicit the inflammatory responses that are associated with necrosis, though the reasons are not clear. Cell death by apoptosis has been noted in cell studies, particularly in relation to abnormal intracellular retention of mutated proteins. Misfolding of the rod visual pigment Rhodopsin has been discovered that prevents its transportation to the outer segment. Dysfunction of cell transport systems can also occur that are involved with photoreceptor protein localization. RP1 was recently found to be a microtubule-associated protein (MAP) and responsible for the organisation of the photoreceptor outer segment, and disruption of its C-terminal may be responsible for the development of RP (Chiang et al., 2006). Rhodopsin is first synthesized in the inner segments of rod photoreceptor cells, and RP1 plays a role in its transportation to the outer segment. Mutations involving RP1 lead to the mislocalization of Rhodopsin to the inner segment (Gao et al., 2002; Liu et al., 2002). Mutations in the carbonic anhydrase IV gene results in its impaired trafficking to the cell surface, the induction of elevated levels of endoplasmic reticulum (ER) stress markers and apoptotic cell death (Datta et al., 2009). cGMP-dependent protein kinase seems to play a key role in mediating cell death (Paquet-Durand et al., 2009), with its overexpresion in wild-type retina leading to cell death, and its inhibition in mouse models of rd1 and rd2 strongly reducing photoreceptor cell death. Telomere length, that may be related to apoptotic photoreceptor cell death, has been found not to be related to the severity of RP, specifically with regards to the Pro23His rhodopsin mutation, and is therefore not a contributing factor (Hartong et al., 2009).

microRNAs (miRNAs) have been implicated recently in the RP apoptotic process (Xu, 2009). These are endogenous, small, non-coding, regulatory RNAs, approximately 22 nucleotides in size. Since the first discovery of miRNAs in 1993 in Caenorhabditis elegans, miRNAs have been shown to be widely expressed in metazoans and plants in tissue-specific and developmental stage-specific manners. miRNAs target their downstream messenger RNAs (mRNAs) by base pairing to their target sites with sequence complementarity, **mainly in the 3'** untranslated region (UTR), and induce the breakdown of the targeted mRNAs and/or inhibition of translation from the mRNAs. Approximately 30% of the protein coding genes are estimated to be regulated by miRNAs. One miRNA can target hundreds of downstream target mRNAs, while one mRNA can be targeted by multiple miRNAs. miRNAs have been recognized as a major level of post-transcriptional regulation of the fine-tuning of gene expression, playing important roles in cellular proliferation, differentiation, and cell death and are involved in all aspects of the biological processes investigated thus far. Mutations in miRNAs and/or the target sites in the transcripts of their downstream target genes and dysregulation of miRNA biogenesis can result in a wide variety of diseases, including cancers. In Pro347Ser RHO transgenic mice that carry a transgene of a mutant form of rhodopsin with the dominant RP mutation, Pro347Ser, it has been found that expression of miR-96 and miR-183 was decreased by 2.5 fold, and miR-1 and miR-133 was increased by threefold in the retinas of 1-month-old Pro347Ser RHO transgenic mice when compared to the ones of wild type controls (Loscher et al., 2007), suggesting that these miRNAs may be involved in the progression of pathological changes in the retinas of this transgenic RP mouse model. It has been suggested that upregulation of miR-1 and miR-133 may repress the expression of an apoptosis inhibitor gene, Fas apoptotic inhibitor molecule (FAIM), and contributes to the apoptosis in the defective photoreceptors. These changes in miRNA levels do not seem to be specific to type of mutation or to the type of inheritance, either dominant or recessive (Loscher et al., 2008).

Therapies Currently being Investigated

No effective therapy exists at present. However, several laboratories are looking at curing the disease from many different angles, or at least slowing it down, using both invasive and non-invasive techniques. Stem cells have been induced to differentiate into a broad range of cell types including photoreceptors and neurons. Sub-retinal transplantation of neural progenitor cells has resulted in repopulation of damaged retinas, the growth again of neuronal axons into the optic nerve head and retardation of further retinal degeneration (Snyder et al., 1997; Ahmad I et al., 1999; Chacko et al., 2000;

Young MJ et al., 2000; Mooney and LaMottte, 2008). Other stem cells, this time autologous bone marrow-derived lineage-negative hematopoietic, have been used to reverse the loss of retinal vasculature by incorporating into degenerating blood vessels in two murine models (Smith, 2004). The loss of retinal vasculature is a presumed metabolic consequence of photoreceptor degeneration, and the use of autologous bone marrow has been shown to prevent cone loss. Gene therapy is being considered as another option. In relation to defects in the photoreceptor-specific gene encoding aryl hydrocarbon receptor-interacting protein-like 1 (AIPL1), which can result in juvenile RP, the use of mouse models has shown that photoreceptor cells can be preserved and cellular function restored (Tan et al., 2009). The injection of a rod-derived cone viability factor (RdCVF), which has been found to increase cone survival, induced an increase in cone cell number and a further increase in the corresponding FERG (Yang et al., 2009). Another idea proposed is the bolstering of the endogenous antioxidant defence system as a gene-based treatment strategy for RP (Usui et al., 2009) by inducing the coexpression of superoxide dismutase 2 and Catalase. The use of this method in mice models resulted in a greater cone density compared to controls. In cases where the mutation involves an enzyme, such as carbonic anhydrase IV, the treatment of the cells with its inhibitor, in this case dorzalamide, reduces apoptotic cell death (Datta et al., 2009). Inhibition of cGMP-dependent protein kinase also appears to increase photoreceptor survival in animal models of RP (Paquet-Durand et al., 2009). The use of retinoids, which are a class of keratolytic drugs derived from retinoic acid (and used for treatment of severe acne and psoriasis) act as pharmacological chaperones to promote the correct folding of rhodopsin proteins that misfold due to mutations (Mendes and Cheetham, 2008). Chaperones in general are cytoplasmic proteins of both prokaryotes and eukaryotes that bind to nascent or unfolded polypeptides and ensure correct folding or transport. Chaperone proteins do not covalently bind to their targets and do not form part of the finished product. Hyperbaric oxygen therapy (HBO) has also been tried with reportedly good results (Vingolo et al., 2008). This was a single-centre, comparative, longitudinal case-controlled randomized clinical trial lasting 10 years. Visual acuity was reported to have been maintained longer with HBO therapy with better FERG b-wave responses at the end of the study. Electrical stimulation of the inner nuclear layer has been shown to reduce apoptosis by 20% in adult Royal College of Surgeons rats after 1 day of continuous stimulation (Schmid et al., 2009). The authors explain that this is clinically applicable to humans and may be used in

RP, as neurons in the inner retina like bipolar cells are accessible to electrical stimulation by a retinal implant for the restoration of vision to blind individuals with diseases of the outer retina.

Future Prospects

Retinitis Pigmentosa as noted above is currently untreatable, and a significant contributing factor to this is gaps in our knowledge with respect to the complete mechanism of light transduction, and the development of photoreceptors. However, an analysis of the mutations that cause RP is promoting further research in this area, and it is expected that in the near future, this will be rectified. Ideas for therapy are also increasing exponentially, with many of them having been developed in the last five years. Therefore, a therapeutic option is expected very soon.

Acknowledgments

The author wishes to thank Maria Ellina for her help in finding related published manuscripts.

References

Ahmad, I; Dooley, CM; Thoreson, WB; Rogers, JA; Afiat, S. In vitro analysis of a mammalian retinal progenitor that gives rise to neurons and glia. *Brain Res.*, 1999, 831, 1-2.

Aleman, TS; Cideciyan, AV; Sumaroka, A; Windsor, EAM; Herrera, W; White, DA; Kaushal, S; Naidu, A; Roman, AJ; Schwartz, SB; Stone, EM; Jacobson, SG. Retinal laminar architecture in human retinitis pigmentosa caused by rhodopsin gene mutations. *Investig Ophthalmol Vis Sci.*, 2008, 49, 1580-1590.

Aleman, TS; Lam, BL; Cideciyan, AV; Sumaroka, A; Windsor, EAM; Roman, AJ; Schwartz, SB; Stone, EM; Jacobson, SG. Genetic heterogeneity in autosomal dominant retinitis pigmentosa with low-frequency damped electroretinographic wavelets. *Eye.*, 2009, 23, 230-233.

Alexander, KR; Rajagopalan, AS; Seiple, W; Zemon, VM; Fishman, GA. Contrast response properties of magnocellular and parvocellular pathways in retinitis pigmentosa assessed by the visual evoked potential. *Investig Ophthalmol Vis Sci.*, 2005, 46, 2967-2973.

Al-Maghtheh, M; Gregory, C; Inglehearn, C; Hardcastle, A; Bhattacharya, S. Rhodopsin mutations in autosomal dominant retinitis pigmentosa. *Hum Mut.*, 1993, 2, 249-255.

Bach, M; Hawlina, M; Holder, GE; Marmor, MF; Meigen, T; Vaegen Miyake, Y. Standard for Pattern Electroretinography. In: Principles and practice of clinical electrophysiology of vision. Heckenlively JR and Arden GB (editors). *MIT Press Bookes.*, 2006, 297-300.

Bhatti, MT. Retinitis pigmentosa, pigmentary retinopathies, and neurologic diseases. *Curr Neurol Neurosci Rep.*, 2006, 6, 403-413.

Birch, DG; Wesley, KH; deFaller, JM; Disbrow, DT; Birch, EE. The relationship between rod perimetric thresholds and full-field rod ERGs in retinits pigmentosa. *Invest Ophthalmol Vis Sci.*, 1987, 28, 954-965.

Birch, DG. Retinitis Pigmentosa. In: Principles and practice of clinical electrophysiology of vision. J. R. Heckenlively, & G. B. Arden (Eds.), *MIT Press Bookes.*, 781-794, 2006.

Bowne, SJ; Liu, Q; Sullivan, LS; Zhu, J; Spellicy, CJ; Rickman, CB; Pierce, EA; Daiger, SP. Why do mutations in the ubiquitously expressed housekeeping gene IMPDH1 cause retina-specific photoreceptor degeneration? *Invest Ophthalmol Vis Sci.*, 2006, 47, 3754-3765.

Bunker, CH; Berson, EL; Bromley, WC; Hayes, RP; Roderick, TH, Prevalence of retinitis pigmentosa in Maine. *Am J Ophthalmol.*, 1984, 97, 357-365.

Celesia, GG; Bodis-Wollner, I; Chatrian, GE; Harding, GFA; Sokol, S; Spekreijse, H. Recommended standards for electroretinograms and visual evoked potentials. Report of an IFCN committee. *Electroencephalogr Clin Neurophysiol.*, 1993, 87, 421-436.

Chacko, DM; Rogers, JA; Turner, JE; Ahmad, I. Survival and differentiation of cultured retinal progenitors transplanted in the subretinal space of the rat. *Biochem Biophys Res Commun.*, 2000, 268, 842-846.

Chiang, SWY; Wang, DY; Chan, WM; Tam, PO; Chong, KK; Lam, DS; Pang, CP. A novel missense RP1 mutation in retinitis pigmentosa. *Eye.*, 2006, 20, 602-605.

Chiappa, KH; Hill, RA. Pattern-shift visual evoked potentials: Interpretation. *In: Evoked potentials in clinical medicine, third edition*, Chiappa KH (editor), Lippincott-Raven publication, 1997, 95-130.

Chiappa, KH. Principles of evoked potentials. In: *Evoked potentials in clinical medicine, third edition*, K. H. Chiappa (Editor), Lippincott-Raven publication, 1997, 1-30.

Datta, R; Waheed, A; Bonapace, G; Shah, GN; Sly, WS. Pathogenesis of retinitis pigmentosa associated with apoptosis-inducing mutations in carbonic anhydrase IV. *Proc Natl Acad Sci.*, U.S.A., 2009, 106, 3437-3442.

Donders, FC. Beitrage zur pathologischen anatomie des auges; 2) Pigmentbildung in der netzhaut. *Graefes Arch Ophthalmol.*, 1857, 3, 138-150.

Dryja, TP; McGee, TL; Hahn, LB; Cowley, GS; Olsson, JE; Reichel, E; Sandberg, MA; Berson, EL. Mutations within the rhodopsin gene in patients with autosomal dominant retinitis pigmentosa. *N Engl J Med.*, 1990, 323, 1302-1307.

Dyrja, TP; Finn, JT; Peng, Y-W; McGee, TL; Berson, EL; Yau, KW. Mutations in the gene encoding the α subunit of the rod cGMP-gated channel in autosomal recessive retinitis pigmentosa. *Proc Natl Acad Sci.*, 1995, 92, 10177-10181.

Farjo, R; Naash, MI. The role of Rds in outer segment morphogenesis and human retinal disease. *Ophthalmic Genet.*, 2006, 27, 117-122.

Farrer, GJ; McWilliam, P; Bradley, DG; Kenna, P; Lawler, M; Sharp, EM, Humphries, MM; Eiberg, H; Conneally, PM; Trofatter, JA. Autosomal dominant retinitis pigmentosa: Linkage to rhodopsin and evidence for genetic heterogeneity. *Genomics*, 1990, 8, 35-40.

Flannery, JG; Farber, DB; Bird, AC; Bok, D. Degenerative changes in a retina affected with autosomal dominant retinitis pigmentosa. *Invest Ophthalmol Vis Sci.*, 1989, 30, 191-211.

Goodwin, P. Hereditary retinal disease. *Curr Opin Ophthalmol.*, 2008, 19, 255-262.

Grover, S; Fishman, GA; Alexander, KR; Anderson, RJ; Derlacki, DJ. Visual acuity impairement in patients with retinitis pigmentosa. *Ophthalomol.*, 1996, 103, 1593-1600.

Hajali, M; Fishman, GA. The prevalence of cystoid macular oedema on optical coherence tomography in retinitis pigmentosa patients without cystic changes on fundus examination. *Eye.*, 2008, doi, 10.1038/eye.2008.110.

Hartong, DT; McGee, TL; Sandberg, MA; Berson, EL; Asselbergs, FW; van der Harst, P; De Vivo, I; Dryja, TP. Search for a correlation between telomere length and severity of retinitis pigmentosa due to the dominant rhodopsin Pro23His mutation. *Mol Vis.*, 2009, 15, 592-597.

He, S; Parapuram, SK; Hurd, TW; Behnam, B; Margolis, B; Swaroop, A, Khanna, H. Retinitis pigmentosa GTPase regulator (RPGR) protein isoforms in mammalian retina: Insights into X-linked retinitis pigmentosa and associated ciliopathies. *Vis Res.*, 2008, 48, 366-376.

Hong, DH; Pawlyk, BS; Shang, J; Sandberg, MA; Berson, EL; Li, T. A retinitis pigmentosa GTPase regulator (RPGR)- deficient mouse model for X-linked retinitis pigmentosa (RP3). *Proc Natl Acad Sci.*, U. S. A., 2000, 97, 3649-3654.

Hood, DC; Lin, CE; Lazow, MA; Locke, KG; Zhang, X; Birch, DG. Thickness of receptor and post-receptor retinal layers in patients with retinitis pigmentosa measured with frequency-domain optical coherence tomography (fdOCT). *Invest Ophthalmol Vis Sci.*, 2008 Nov 14 [Epub ahead of print].

Humayun, MS; Prince, M; de Juan, E Jr.; Barron, Y; Moskowitz, M; Klock, IB; Milam, AH. Morphometric analysis of the extramacular retina from post-mortem eyes with retinitis pigmentosa. *Invest Ophthalmol Vis Sci.*, 1999, 40, 143-148.

Humbert, G; Delettre, C; Sénéchal, A; Bazalgette, C; Barakat, A; Bazalgette, C; Arnaud, B; Lenaers, G; Hamel, CP. Homozygous deletion related to Alu repeats in RLBP1 causes retinitis pigmentosa albescens. *Invest Ophthalmol Vis Sci.*, 2006, 47, 4719-4724.

Huranová, M; Hnilicová, J; Fleischer, B; Cvacová, Z; Stanek, D. A mutation linked to retinitis pigmentosa in HPRP31 causes proteint instability and impairs its interactions with spliceosomal snRNPs. *Hum Mol Gen.*, 2009, Mar 17 [Epub ahead of print].

Janaky, M; Palffy, A; Horvath, G; Tuboly, G; Benedek, G. Pattern-reversal electroretinograms and visual evoked potentials in retinitis pigmentosa. *Doc Opthalmol.*, 2008, 117, 27-36.

Kriss, A; Jeffrey, B; Taylor, D. The electroretinogram in infants and young children. 1992, 9, 373-393.

Lam, BL; Liu, M; Hamasaki, DI. Low-frequency damped electroretinographic wavelets in young asymptomatic patients with dominant retinitis pigmentosa: a new electroretinographic finding. *Ophthalmol.*, 1999, 106, 1109–1113.

Liu, Q; Zhou, J; Daiger, SP; Farber, DB; Heckenlively, JR; Smith, JE; Sullivan, LS; Zuo, J; Milam, AH; Pierce, EA. Identification and subcellular localization of the RP1 protein in human and mouse photoreceptor. *Invest Ophthalmol Vis Sci.*, 2002, 43, 22-23.

Loscher, CJ; Hokamp, K; Kenna, PF; Ivens, AC; Humphries, P; Palfi, A; Farrar, GJ. Altered retinal microRNA expression profile in a mouse model of retinitis pigmentosa. *Genome Biol.*, 2007, 8, R248.

Loscher, CJ; Hokamp, K; Wilson, JH; Li, T; Humphries, P; Farrar, GJ; Palfi, A. A common microRNA signature in mouse models of retinal degeneration. *Exp Eye Res.*, 2008, 87, 529-534.

Lyon, MF; (1961) Gene action in the x-chromosome of the mouse. *Nature.*, 190, 372-373

Marmor, MF; Hood, DC; Keating, D; Kondo, M; Seeliger, MW; Miyake, Y. Guidelines for basic multifocal electroretinography (mfERG). In: Principles and practice of clinical electrophysiology of vision. Heckenlively JR and Arden GB (editors). *MIT Press Bookes.*, 309-318, 2006.

Mendes, HF; Cheetham, ME. Pharmacological manipulations of gain-of-function and dominant-negative mechanisms in rhodopsin retinitis pigmentosa. *Hum Mol Genet.*, 2008, 17, 3043-3054.

Mendes, HF; van der Spuy, J; Chapple, JP; Cheetman, ME. Mechanisms of cell death in rhodopsin retinitis pigmentosa: implications for therapy. *Trends in Molecular Medicine.*, 2005, 11, 177-185.

Milam, AH; Li, ZY; Fariss, RN. Histopathology of the human retina in retinitis pigmentosa. *Prog Retin Eye Res.*, 1998, 17, 175-205.

Mooney, I; LaMotte, J. A review of the potential to restore vision with stem cells. *Clin Exp Optom.*, 2008, 91, 78-84.

Morimura, H; Berson, EL; Dryja, TP. Recessive mutations in the RLBP1 gene encoding cellular retinaldehyde-binding protein in a form of retinitis punctata albescens. *Invest Ophthalmol Vis Sci.*, 1999, 40, 1000-1004.

Nagy, D; Schönfisch, B; Zrenner, E; Jägle, H. Long-term follow-up of retinitis pigmentosa patients with multifocal electroretinography. *Invest Ophthalmol Vis Sci.*, 2008, 49, 4664-4671.

Neidhardt, J; Glaus, E; Lorenz, B; Netzer, C; Li, Y; Schambeck, M; Wittmer, M; Feil, S; Kirschner-Schwabe, R; Rosenberg T, Cremers, FPM; Bergen, AAB; Barthelmes, D; Baraki, H; Schmid, F; Tanner, G; Fleischhauer, J; Orth, U; Becker, C; Wegscheider, E; Nürnberg, G; Nürnberg, P; Bolz, HJ; Gal, A; Berger, W. Identification of novel mutations in X-linked retinitis pigmentosa families and implications for diagnostic testing. *Mol Vis.*, 2008, 14, 1081-1093.

Newman, NM; Stevens, RA; Heckenlively, JR. Nerve fibre layer loss in diseases of the outer retinal layer. *Br J Ophthalmol.*, 1987, 71, 21-26.

Odom, JV; Bach, M; Barber, C; Brigell, M; Marmor, MF; Tormene, AP; Holder, GE; Vaegen. Visual evoked potentials standard (2004). *Doc Ophthalmol.*, 2004, 108, 115-123.

Oishi, A; Otani, A; Sasahara, M; Kurimoto, M; Nakamura, H; Kojima, H; Yoshimura, N. Retinal nerve fiber layer thickness in patients with retinitis pigmentosa. *Eye.*, 2009, 23, 561-566.

Papathanasiou, ES; Papacostas, SS. Flash electroretinography: normative values with surface skin electrodes and no pupil dilation using a standard stimulation protocol. *Doc Ophthalmol.*, 2008, 116, 61-73.

Paquet-Durand, F; Hauck, SM; van Veen, T; Ueffing, M; Ekström, P. PKG activity causes photoreceptor cell death in two retinitis pigmentosa models. *J Neurochem.*, 2009, 108, 796-810.

Paranhos, FR; Katsum, O; Arai, M; Nehemy, MB; Hirose, T. Pattern reversal visual evoked response in retinitis pigmentosa. *Doc Ophthalmol.*, 1998-1999, 96, 321-331.

Pimkin, M; Pimkina, J; Markham, GD. A regulatory role of the Bateman domain of IMP dehydrogenase in adenylate nucleotide biosynthesis. *J Biol Chem.*, 2009, 284, 7960-7969.

Rehemtulla, A; Warwar, R; Kumar, R; Ji, X; Zack, DJ; Swaroop, A. The basic motif-leucine zipper transcription factor Nrl can positively regulate rhodopsin gene expression. *Proc Natl Acad Sci.*, USA., 1996, 93, 191-195.

Rousseff, RT; Tzvetanov, P; Rousseva, MA. The bifid visual evoked potential-normal variant or a sign of demyelination. *Clin Neurophysiol.*, 2005, 107, 113-116.

Sakata, LM; Deleon-Ortega, J; Sakata, V; Girkin, CA. Optic coherence tomography of the retina and optic nerve-a review. *Clin Experiment Ophthalmol.*, 2009, 37, 90-99.

Sancho-Pelluz, J; Arango-Gonzalez, B; Kustermann, S; Romero, FJ; van Veen, T; Zrenner, E; Ekström, P; Paquet-Durand, F. Photoreceptor cell death mechanisms in inherited retinal degeneration. *Mol Neurobiol.*, 2008, 38, 253-269.

Sandberg, MA; Brockhurst, RJ; Gaudio, AR; Berson, EL. Visual acuity is related to parafoveal retinal thickness in patients with retinitis pigmentosa and macular cysts. Invest. *Ophthalmol Vis Sci.*, 2008, 49, 4568-4572.

Sandberg, MA; Rosner, B; Weigel-DiFranco, C; McGee, TL; Dryja, TP; Berson, EL. Disease course in patients with autosomal recessive retinitis pigmentosa due to the USH2A gene. *Invest Ophthalmol Vis Sci.*, 2008, 49, 5532-5539.

Sandberg, MA; Weigel-DiFranco, C; Rosner, B; Berson, EL. The relationship between visual field size and electroretinogram amplitude in Retinitis Pigmentosa. *Invest Ophthalmol Vis Sci.*, 1996, 37, 1693-1698.

Santos, A; Humayun, MS; de Juan, EJ; Greenburg, RJ; Marsh, MJ; Klock, IB; Milam, AH. Preservation of the inner retina in retinitis pigmentosa: a morphometric analysis. *Arch Ophthalmol.*, 1997, 115, 511-515.

Schmid, H; Herrman, T; Kohler, K; Stett, A. Neuroprotective effect of transretinal electrical stimulation on neurons in the inner nuclear layer of the degenerated retina. *Brain Res Bull.*, 2009, 79, 15-25.

Seiple, W; Clemens, CJ; Greenstein, VC; Carr, RE; Holopigian, K. Test–retest reliability of the multifocal electroretinogram and Humphrey visual fields in patients with retinitis pigmentosa. *Doc Ophthalmol.*, 2004, 109, 255-272.

Shastry, BS. Retinitis pigmentosa and related disorders: phenotypes of rhodopsin and peripherin/RDS mutations. *Am J Med Genet.*, 1994, 52, 467-474.

Smith, LE. Bone marrow-derived stem cells preserve cone vision in retinitis pigmentosa. *J Clin Invest.*, 2004, 114, 755-757.

Snyder, EY; Yoon, C; Flax, JD; Macklis, JD. Multipotent neural precursors can differentiate toward replacement of neurons undergoing targeted apoptotic degeneration in adult mouse neocortex. *Proc Nat Acad Sci.*, USA, 1997, 94, 11663-11668.

Stone, JL; Barlow, WE; Humayun, MS; de Juan, E; Milam, AH. Morphometric analysis of macular photoreceptors and ganglion cells in retinas with retinitis pigmentosa. *Arch Ophthalomol.*, 1992, 110, 1634-1639.

Sugawara, T; Hagiwara, A; Hiramatsu, A; Ogata, K; Mitamura, Y; Yamamoto, S. Relationship between peripheral visual field loss and vision-related quality of life in patients with retinitis pigmentosa. *Eye.*, 2009, doi: 10.1038/eye.2009.176.

Sun, XC; Li, J; Cui, M; Bonanno, JA. Role of carbonic anhydrase IV in corneal endothelial NCO_3^- transport. *Investig Ophthalmol Vis Sci.*, 2008, 49, 1048-1055.

Tam, LC; Kiang, AS; Kennan, A; Kenna, PF; Chadderton, N; Ader, N; Palfi, A; Aherne, A; Ayuso, C; Campbell, M; Reynolds, A; McKee, A; Humphries, MM; Farrar, GL; Humphries, P. Therapeutic benefit derived from RNAi-mediated ablation of IMPDH1 transcripts in a murine model of autosomal dominant retinitis pigmentosa (RP10). *Hum Mol Genet.*, 2008, 17, 2084-2100.

Tan, MH; Smith, AJ; Pawlyk, B; Xu, X; Liu, X; Bainbridge, JB; Basche, M; McIntosh, J; Tran, HV; Nathwani, A; Li, T; Ali, RR. Gene therapy for retinitis pigmentosa and Leber congenital amaurosis caused by defects in AIPL1: effective rescue of mouse models of partial and complete aipl1 deficiency using AAV2/2 and AAV2/8 vectors. *Hum Mol Genet.*, 2009, Mar 19 [Epub ahead of print].

Tuson, M; Garanto, A; Gonzàlez-Duarte, R; Marfany, G. Overexpression of CERKL, a gene responsible for retinitis pigmentosa in humans, protects cells from apoptosis induced by oxidative stress. *Mol Vis.*, 2009, 15, 168-180.

Usui, S; Komeima, K; Lee, SY; Jo, YJ; Ueno, S; Rogers, BS; Wu, Z; Shen, J; Lu, L; Oveson, BC; Rabinovitch, PS; Campochiaro, PA. Increased expression of Catalase and Superoxide Dismutase 2 reduces cone cell death in retinitis pigmentosa. *Mol Ther.*, 2009 [Epub ahead of print].

Vajaranant, TS; Seiple, W; Szlyk, JP; Fishman, GA. Detection using the multifocal electroretinogram of mosaic retinal dysfunction in carriers of X-linked retinitis pigmentosa. *Ophthalmol*, 2002, 109, 560-568.

Van Nie, R; Ivanyi, D; Demant, P. A new H-2-linked mutation, rds, causing retinal degeneration in the mouse. *Tiss Ant.*, 1978, 12, 106-108.

Vingolo, EM; Livani, ML; Domanico, D; Mendonça, RHF; Rispoli, E. Optical coherence tomography and electro-oculogram abnormalities in X-linked retinitis pigmentosa. *Doc Ophthalmol.*, 2006, 113, 5-10.

Vingolo, EM; Rocco, M; Grenga, P; Salvatore, S; Pelaia, P. Slowing the degenerative process, long lasting effect of hyperbaric oxygen therapy in retinitis pigmentosa. *Graefes Arch Clin Exp Ophthalmol.*, 2008, 246, 93-98.

Vingolo, EM; Salvatore, S; Stagnitti, F. Visual acuity changes in retinitis pigmentosa during pregnancy. *Int J Gyn Obstet.*, 2009, doi, 10.1016/j.ijgo.2009.01.027.

Walia, S; Fishman, GA; Edward, DP; Lindeman, M. Retinal nerve fiber layer defects in RP patients. *Investig Ophthalmol Vis Sci.*, 2007, 48, 4748-4752.

Wang, H; den Hollander, AI; Moayedi, Y; Abulimiti, A; Li, Y; Collin, RWJ; Hoyng, CB; Lopez, I; Brag, M; Lewis, RA; Lupski, JR; Mardon, G; Koenekoop, RK; Chen, R. Mutations in SPATA7 cause Leber Congenital

Amaurosis and Juvenile Retinitis Pigmentosa. *Am J Hum Gen.*, 2009, 84, 380-387.

Weinstein, GW; Odom, JV; Cavender, S. Visually evoked potentials and electroretinography in neurological evaluation. *Neurol Clin.*, 1991, 9, 225-242.

Xu, S. microRNA expression in the eyes and their significance in relation to functions. *Prog Retin Eye Res.*, 2009, 28, 87-116.

Yagasaki, K; Jacobson, SG; Apathy, PP; Knighton, RW. Rod and cone psychophysics and electroretinography: Methods for comparison in retinal degenerations. *Doc Ophthalmol.*, 1988, 69, 119-130.

Yang, Y; Mohand-Said, S; Danan, A; Simonutti, M; Fontaine, V; Clerin, E; Picaud, S; Léveillard, T; Sahel, JA. Functional cone rescue by RdCVF protein in a dominant model of retinitis pigmentosa. *Mol Ther.*, 2009, Mar 20 [Epub ahead of print].

Yang-Feng, TL; Swaroop, A. Neural retina-specific leucine zipper gene NRL (D14S46E) maps to human chromosome 14q11.1-q11.2. *Genomics*, 1992, 14, 491-492.

Yoon, JH; Qiu, J; Cai, S; Chen, Y; Cheetham, ME; Shen, B; Pfeifer, GP. The retinitis pigmentosa-mutated RP2 protein exhibits exonuclease activity and translocates to the nucleus in response to DNA damage. *Exp Cell Res.*, 2006, 312, 1323-1334.

Young, MJ; Ray, J; Whiteley, SJO; Klassen, H; Gage, F. Neuronal differentiation and morphological integration of hippocampal progenitor cells transplanted to the retina of immature and mature dystrophic rats. *Mol Cell Neurosci.*, 2000, 16, 197-205.

In: Reginitis Pigmentosa: Causes, Diagnosis...   ISBN: 978-1-60876-884-4
Editors: M. Baert, et al. pp. 89-110   © 2010 Nova Science Publishers, Inc.

Chapter III

Great Expectations: *RPE65* Mutations in South Africa

Lisa Roberts, George Rebello,
Jacquie Greenberg and Raj Ramesar
MRC Human Genetics Research Unit, Division of Human Genetics,
Department of Clinical Laboratory Sciences, Institute of Infectious Disease
and Molecular Medicine, Faculty of Health Sciences,
University of Cape Town, South Africa.

Abstract

Recently, *RPE65* gene replacement therapy in a total of nine human subjects with Leber congenital amaurosis marked the first treatment for genetic retinal degenerative diseases (RDD). The prospect of imminent gene therapy made *RPE65* a strong candidate for mutation screening in South Africa. An added impetus for this study was the fact that a founder mutation in *RPE65* was described as causing an early onset RDD in an isolated Dutch population, and the founder effect in South Africans descended from Dutch settlers has been well documented for other diseases and genes.

Mutations in the *RPE65* gene are reported to be responsible for approximately 2% of autosomal recessive retinitis pigmentosa (arRP) and 16% of Leber congenital amaurosis (LCA). For this study a cohort of 87 affected, unrelated individuals was selected for mutation screening. Of these individuals, 18 were classified as having LCA and 69 as having early onset RP (with an age of onset younger than 15 years). Of the LCA cohort, 4 exhibited autosomal recessive inheritance (arLCA) and 14 were isolated cases. Of the RP cohort, 44 had arRP and 25 were isolated cases. The ethnic breakdown of the cohort was as follows: 65 were Caucasian, 7 were indigenous Black African, 10 of Asian Indian origin, 4 of Mixed Ancestry (comprising individuals whose ancestry is a mixture of Caucasian, Malaysian, Madagascan and indigenous African including Khoi-San and West African) and 1 was Taiwanese. The 14 exons of *RPE65*, including the intron/exon boundaries, were screened using denaturing high performance liquid chromatography (dHPLC) analysis and variations were characterised by direct sequencing.

Five different pathogenic mutations (of which 2 were novel) were identified in the cohort of 69 individuals diagnosed with early onset RP. The Dutch founder mutation, Tyr368His, was the only homozygous mutation detected and was identified in a family of Mixed Ancestry with arRP. In two families, compound heterozygous mutations in *RPE65* are presumed to be causative of disease: Ala132Thr and the novel IVS1+1G>T mutation was present in one Indian family with arRP; Leu22Pro and the novel Glu21Lys mutation were present in one Caucasian individual with isolated RP. In two cases (one Indian family with arRP and one Caucasian individual with isolated RP) a single heterozygous Ala132Thr mutation was identified and the second mutation, should it exist, is unknown. This Ala132Thr mutation was the single most common variation detected, as it was identified in three of the 69 individuals classified as having RP (4.4%). No pathogenic mutations were identified in the cohort of patients diagnosed with LCA.

The identification of disease-causing genetic mutations in families with RDD generally means that predictive, diagnostic and prenatal testing can be offered to family members, although few options exist for treatment. Importantly, three families in South Africa possibly stand to benefit from therapeutic intervention by *RPE65* gene replacement therapy.

Introduction

The gene encoding the retinal pigment epithelium-specific protein 65kDa (*RPE65*) was characterised in 1995 [1]. This gene, which is expressed in the retinal pigment epithelium (RPE), produces an isomerohydrolase enzyme that catalyses an important stage of the visual retinoid cycle [2]. In the visual transduction pathway, the 11-*cis* retinal chromophore of rhodopsin is isomerised to all-*trans* retinal. Regeneration of 11-*cis* retinal and the consequent regeneration of rhodopsin, via the visual retinoid cycle, are essential for visual function. RPE65 functions to convert all-trans retinyl ester to 11-cis retinol. Loss of *RPE65* function in mice has been observed to result in deficiencies of 11-*cis* retinal and functional rhodopsin, as well as an accumulation of opsin and all-*trans* retinal ester [3, 4].

In humans, mutations of the *RPE65* gene are reportedly responsible for approximately 2% of autosomal recessive retinitis pigmentosa (arRP) and 16% of Leber congenital amaurosis (LCA) [5]. LCA is a group of recessively inherited rod-cone dystrophies that result in bilateral vision loss in childhood [6]. RP is a group of retinal degenerative diseases (RDD) characterised by nightblindness, progressive loss of peripheral visual fields and eventual loss of central vision. The most prevalent form of RP is arRP, some of the symptoms of which often overlap with LCA [7]. Modifier effects have also been identified, with the Leu450Met *RPE65* variant reportedly protecting against light damage and reducing retinal degeneration through the modulation of rhodopsin regeneration [8-10].

The vision loss associated with *RPE65* mutations is initially biochemical. The RPE itself remains intact, although degeneration of the photoreceptors eventually occurs as a secondary event. The lack of immediate photoreceptor degeneration in LCA made *RPE65* an excellent candidate for gene therapy. Several studies have shown that wild-type gene delivery generates isomerohydrolase activity and restores vision in canine and murine models with this disease phenotype [11-15] . In 2001, wild-type *RPE65* in an adeno-associated viral vector restored vision when injected subretinally into the eye of an LCA canine [11]. In 2005, the same group reported that a single treatment restored vision in approximately 89% of canine eyes, that the response remained stable after 3 years, and that no deleterious effects were observed [12]. In 2005, patients with LCA due to *RPE65* mutations were identified by clinical and molecular profiling and recruited for a Phase I trial to assess treatment safety [15]. In 2008, the results of three clinical trials, each treating three young adults, were published [16-18]. The results of these trials are difficult to combine and interpret, as many parameters were dissimilar; including the regulatory elements controlling expression of the human *RPE65* in the adeno-associated viral vectors, and the level of visual function of the nine patients prior to treatment. However, no systemic toxicity or immune response post-treatment was observed in any of the trial participants and improved efficacy may be obtained in the future through the optimisation of doses, refinement of microsurgery techniques and treatment of LCA patients retaining greater baseline visual function.

South Africa (SA) has a rich immigrant history, with contributions notably from Great Britain, the Netherlands, Germany and France in the northern hemisphere, and India and Malaysia in the east [19]. From the genetics perspective, founder effects have been described for a wide range of inherited conditions. The founder effect in South Africans descended from Dutch settlers, specifically, has been reported for other diseases [20, 21]. A founder mutation in *RPE65*, Tyr368His, was previously described as causing an early onset severe retinal dystrophy in an isolated Dutch population in the Netherlands [22].

The possibility of a founder effect in SA and the imminence of a potential therapy lead to the selection of *RPE65* as a candidate gene for mutation analysis in SA patients with RDD.

Methods

Subjects

Individuals affected with RDD and their family members are referred to the Division of Human Genetics at the University of Cape Town (UCT), from throughout SA. A research program was initiated in 1990 [23] with the ultimate goal of identifying the causative genetic mutation in each of the families registered in the UCT RDD database. Demographic information, biological material and clinical details have been archived for over 1200 families with various RDD.

Informed consent was obtained according to the Declaration of Helsinki (2000), and this research project was approved by the research ethics committee of the Faculty of Health Sciences, University of Cape Town.

It should be noted that a preponderance of Caucasian individuals is observed due to a historical ascertainment bias and the lack of resources in rural areas where the majority of the indigenous populations reside. As a result, the ethnic breakdown of the archived samples does not reflect the population distribution. "Caucasian" refers to people of West European origin, mainly Dutch, French, German and British. "Black African" refers to indigenous people of Black African origin and "Indian" refers to people whose ancestors settled in SA from India. The "Mixed Ancestry" population comprises those whose ancestry is a mixture of Caucasian, Malaysian, Madagascan and Black African (including Khoi-San and West African) [24].

A cohort of 87 affected, unrelated individuals was selected for *RPE65* mutation analysis (Table 1). Of these individuals, 18 were classified as having LCA and 69 as having early onset RP (with an age of onset younger than 15 years). Of the LCA cases, 4 exhibited autosomal recessive inheritance (arLCA) and 14 were isolated cases. Of the RP cases, 44 exhibited autosomal recessive inheritance (arRP) and 25 were isolated cases. The ethic breakdown of the 87 individuals is as follows: 65 Caucasian, 7 Black African, 10 Indian, 4 Mixed Ancestry and 1 Taiwanese. None of the individuals had a causative mutation identified in another gene.

Table 1. The ethnic breakdown of the cohort selected for *RPE65* mutation screening, indicating the number of individuals with each RDD.

Ethnic Group	arLCA	Isolated LCA	arRP	Isolated RP	Total no. of individuals per ethnic group
Caucasian	4	13	31	17	65
Black African	-	-	2	5	7
Indian	-	-	7	3	10
Mixed Ancestry	-	-	4	-	4
Taiwanese	-	1	-	-	1
Total no. of individuals per RDD	4	14	44	25	87

PCR and Heteroduplex Formation

Primers spanning the entire coding region of *RPE65* were used to amplify the exons and intron/exons boundaries of the gene in each proband (Table 2).

PCR amplification was performed using standard conditions. Thermal cycling conditions for exons 10 and 11-13 were: 95°C - 5 minutes; 30 cycles of {95°C for 30 seconds, T_a°C for 30 seconds, 72°C for 30 seconds}; 72°C for 5 minutes. The T_a of exon 10 and 11-13 were 50°C and 47°C respectively. The following touchdown thermal cycling conditions were used for the remaining exons: 95°C - 3 minutes; 10 cycles with decreasing T_a {94°C for 15 seconds, 60 → 55°C for 15 seconds, 72°C for 30 seconds}; 20 cycles of {89°C for 15 seconds, 55°C for 15 seconds, 72°C for 30 seconds}; 72°C for 5 minutes.

Table 2. The primer sequences used for *RPE65* mutation screening.

Exon	Forward primer (5' → 3')	Reverse primer (5' → 3')
1	GAGAGCTGAAAGCAACTTCTG	ATAGCACATTTATCATGAATCCATG
2	CTATCTCTGCGGACTTTGAGC	GCCAGAGAAGAGAGACTG
3	GGCAGGGATAAGAAGCAATG	CTGAGTTCAGAGGTGAAAAC
4-5	CTGTACGGATTGCTCCTGTC	GAACATCACCTAGCACTGTG
6	TATAATGTATCTTCCTTCTCTCAAC	CTCACAATACAGTAACTTTCTCAC
7-8	AAATAAGAGGCTGTTCCAAAGC	TTAAACACATCTTCTTCAGAATCAC
9	GTACACTTTTTTCCTTTTTAAATGCATC	GTTTTAGATGTGATTCAGATTGAGTG
10	TGCCTGTGCTCATGTTTGAC	TGAGAGAGATGAAACATTCTGG
11-13	GTTTGAATTCTTTCCTGCTCAC	CTAACATACAGAACTGCAGTAAG
14	AGTCAGAAAAAGAAGTCAGGTC	ATTGCTTGCTCAACTCAGTGC

Post PCR, each test sample was mixed with a wild-type sample prior to heteroduplex formation, to ensure the detection of homozygous variants. Heteroduplex formation was promoted by heat denaturing the samples at 95°C for 5 minutes and allowing the tube temperature to reach room temperature gradually over 45 minutes.

dHPLC Analysis

Denaturing high performance liquid chromatography (dHPLC) was performed using the WAVE® Nucleic Acid Fragment Analysis System (Transgenomic Inc, USA). Several injections, each with a different set of parameters was required per amplicon to ensure analysis across the entire fragment. The variable parameters included temperature, gradient duration, amplicon volume injected and use of a time shift. For all amplicons, the flow rate was 1.5ml/minute.

When numerous samples exhibited the same variant dHPLC profiles, one of these samples was selected as a representative and sequenced. The samples with similar dHPLC profiles were tested for the presence of that variant using a "WAVE mixing experiment", wherein an equal volume of the PCR product under question was mixed with that of the sequenced variant sample prior to heteroduplex formation and dHPLC analysis. Lack of additional peaks indicated that sequences of the PCR product being queried and the known sample were identical. All samples with unique aberrant profiles were sequenced.

Sequencing

PCR products were purified using the QIAquick® gel extraction kit, QIAquick® PCR purification kit or the QIAEX II gel extraction protocol (Qiagen, UK), according to the manufacturer's **instructions**. Purified samples were sequenced using the same forward or reverse primers used for the original PCR. Sequencing reactions were performed using the BigDye® terminator cycle sequencing kit version 3.1 (Applied Biosystems, USA) and one of the following cycling conditions:

- 96°C for 1 min; 25 cycles of {95°C for 45 sec, 60°C for 4 min}
- 96°C for 5 min; 25 cycles of {96°C for 30 sec, 50°C for 15 sec, 60°C for 4 min}

Sequencing products were purified using Centri-Sep columns (Princeton Separations, USA) according to manufacturer's **instructions,** and resolved on an ABI Prism™ 3100 automated sequencer (Applied Biosystems, USA).

Variant Analysis

Novel sequence variants (those which, to the best of our knowledge, had not been previously reported) were analysed to determine whether they were pathogenic or nonpathogenic; restriction enzymes digests were used for familial cosegregation analyses and to screen for a particular variant in 50 controls (100 chromosomes). The control cohorts were ethnically matched to the test sample in which the variant had originally been detected. The control individuals had not been assessed specifically for the presence of RDD. Variants occurring in more than 1% of the alleles in a population were considered unlikely to be pathogenic [25]. Restriction Enzyme digests were performed according to manufacturer's **instructions**. Intronic variants and silent polymorphisms were analysed using version NNSPLICE 0.9 of the

Berkeley Drosophila **Genome Project's splice site prediction** by neural network [26, 27], to determine whether an effect on splicing could be predicted.

Results

A total of 16 different sequence variants were detected in *RPE65*, of which five were determined to be pathogenic (Table 3). Two novel pathogenic mutations, five novel non-pathogenic polymorphisms and one novel variant of unknown pathogenicity were identified in the South African cohort.

Polymorphisms

Eleven variations were detected during mutation screening, and were classified as nonpathogenic polymorphisms. None of the variations were predicted to have any effect on splicing efficiency.

IVS2-18G>A was detected in one sample from the LCA cohort and two samples from the RP cohort. The same two RP samples also carried an IVS3+80T>A variant. Presence of a heterozygous IVS6+22C>T (dbSNP:rs2274321) variant was confirmed in two samples from the LCA cohort and seven samples from the RP cohort. A novel heterozygous c.750C>T variant was identified in one sample from the LCA cohort. This encodes a silent polymorphism, Ile250Ile. The novel IVS7+98C>T was detected in one sample from the RP cohort.

The Asn321Lys variant was detected in the heterozygous state in one Caucasian individual with LCA. The pathogenicity of the variant was previously uncertain as it reportedly occurred in the heterozygous state in a child of a consanguineous marriage and was detected in a control population [28]. A recent study, however, reported that this variant had a low estimate of pathogenic probability due to the fact that it occurred in the heterozygous state on the same allele as a more plausible mutation, was identified in a control cohort, and did not reduce the isomerase function of *RPE65 in vitro* [29]. Subsequent sample analysis using the Asper Biotech Ltd LCA Microarray showed that the disease in the South African individual is due to a homozygous Ser175Arg mutation in the *LRAT* gene.

Table 3. Summary of variations detected in *RPE65*.

Variant	Pathogenic	Novel	Reason variant is described as pathogenic/ nonpathogenic	No. Individuals
IVS1+1G>T	Yes	Yes	Not detected in controls, segregates with disease	1 arRP *(I)*
Glu21Lys	Yes	Yes	Not detected in controls, segregates with disease	1 isolated RP *(C)*
Leu22Pro	Yes	No	Previously reported	1 isolated RP *(C)*
Ala132Thr	Yes	No	Previously reported	2 arRP *(I)*, 1 isolated RP *(C)*
Tyr368His	Yes	No	Previously reported	1 arRP *(M)*
Tyr249Cys	Unknown	Yes	Evolutionary conserved, predicted protein effect, but in-phase with reported mutation	1 arRP *(I)*
IVS2-18G>A	No	Yes	Computational evidence	1 isolated LCA *(C)*, 1 arRP *(C)*, 1 isolated RP *(B)*
IVS3+80T>A	No	Yes	Computational evidence	1 arRP *(C)*, 1 isolated RP *(B)*
IVS6+22C>T	No	No	Previously reported, computational evidence	1 arLCA *(C)*, 1 isolated LCA *(C)*, 3 arRP *(2C,1 I)*, 4 isolated RP *(2C, 1B, 1 I)*
Ile250Ile	No	Yes	Computational evidence	1 arLCA *(C)*
IVS7+98C>T	No	Yes	Computational evidence	1 arRP *(C)*
Asn321Lys	No	No	Conflicting reports, however the causative mutation in this patient was later identified in another gene.	1 isolated LCA *(C)*
Glu352Glu	No	No	Previously reported, computational evidence	2 isolated LCA *(1C, 1T)*, 14 arRP *(10C, 3I, 1B)*, 5 isolated RP *(4C, 1B)*
IVS11+29G>A	No	Yes	Computational evidence	1 isolated LCA *(C)*, 1 arRP *(C)*
IVS12-39T>C	No	No	Previously reported, computational evidence	1 isolated LCA *(C)*, 1 arRP *(B)*, 4 isolated RP *(B)*
IVS12+20A>C	No	No	Previously reported, computational evidence	1 isolated LCA *(T)*, 4 arRP *(3C, 1I)*
Thr385Thr	No	No	Previously reported, computational evidence	1 arRP *(C)*, 1 isolated RP *(B)*

Key: *(C)* = Caucasian, *(I)* = Indian, *(B)* = Black African, *(M)* = Mixed Ancestry, *(T)* = Taiwanese

Glu352Glu (c.1056G>A; dbSNP:rs12145904) was present in the homozygous state in one Taiwanese individual with LCA (isolated case) and 1 Indian individual with arRP, and in the heterozygous state in one individual with LCA and 18 with RP. Glu352Glu has been previously reported as nonpathogenic and occurring at a frequency of 14% of controls and 15% of patients [5].

The novel IVS11+29G>A, was identified in the heterozygous state in one sample from each cohort. IVS12-39T>C (dbSNP:rs13375676) was present in the heterozygous state in one LCA sample and five RP samples. IVS12+20A>C (dbSNP:rs12564647) was identified in the homozygous state in one LCA sample and heterozygous state in four RP samples including one with IVS11+29G>A. This intronic change was previously reported as nonpathogenic and occurring at a frequency of 4% in control individuals and 3% in patients [5]. An isocoding variant, Thr385Thr (c.1155G>A) was identified in two RP samples, including one with IVS12-39T>C, and has been previously reported as being nonpathogenic [5].

Mutations

Five different mutations were identified in this study, and these mutations were all identified in individuals with RP (Table 4). No mutations were identified in the individuals with LCA.

Table 4: Summary of the families with pathogenic mutations identified in *RPE65*.

Family ID	RDD	Ethnicity	Allele 1	Allele 2
568	arRP	Indian	Ala132Thr (in phase with novel Tyr249Cys)	IVS1+1G>T
387	Isolated RP	Caucasian	Ala132Thr	Unknown
394	arRP	Indian	Ala132Thr	Unknown
373	Isolated RP	Caucasian	Glu21Lys	Leu22Pro
52	arRP	Mixed Ancestry	Tyr368His (Homozygous)	

A heterozygous novel variant IVS1+1G>T, which creates an *Mse I* restriction enzyme site, was detected in one proband with RP, 568.4, and was predicted to abolish the donor splice site of exon 1. A restriction enzyme digest was performed to determine whether the variant co-segregated with disease in family 568, an Indian family. IVS1+1G>T was detected in the heterozygous state in three siblings (two of whom were affected) and the father (Figure 1). DNA from 50 control unaffected Indian individuals was tested for the presence of this variant using the *Mse I* digest. The variation was not detected in the 100 chromosomes tested.

Three samples from RP patients, including 568.4 above, were found to carry a heterozygous Ala132Thr (c.394G>A) mutation, which has previously been reported as causing arRP [5, 28]. The presence of the mutation does not affect a restriction enzyme site, so family studies were performed using the WAVE mixing experiments. In family 568 the Ala132Thr mutation was found to be in-phase with a novel Tyr249Cys (c.746A>G) variant, as both sequence variations were detected in the unaffected mother and each of the two affected siblings, and both sequence variations were absent in the two asymptomatic siblings (Figure 1). Ty249Cys results in a polar amino acid with an aromatic ring being replaced by a nonpolar amino acid which forms disulphide bridges. Protein sequence alignment indicated that the Tyr249 amino acid is conserved in human, mouse, rat, fruit fly, zebra fish, dog, chicken, puffer fish, frog and cow. Although Tyr249Cys may be pathogenic, this could not be confirmed and it would appear that IVS1+1G>T and Ala132Thr are the two causative mutations in family 568.

Of the other RP families in which Ala132Thr was identified, one was also an Indian family (family 394) and the other a Caucasian family (family 387). No second pathogenic mutation was detected in either family (Figure 2).

A dHPLC variation was observed in exon 2 of a proband with RP, 373.1. Sequencing revealed the presence of two heterozygous variations in exon 2 of this individual: the novel Glu21Lys (c.61G>A), and previously reported Leu22Pro (c.65T>C) [30]. Glu21Lys destroys a *Mnl I* restriction enzyme site, and Leu22Pro creates an *NlaIV* site therefore these restriction enzyme digests were performed on samples from two individuals in the family (the affected individual and her mother) (Figure 3). Both variations were present in the affected individual (373.1) and only the Glu21Lys variation was present in the mother (373.2). DNA from 50 control unaffected Caucasian individuals was tested using the *Mnl I* digest and none of these 100 chromosomes were found to carry the variation. This evidence indicates that Glu21Lys is pathogenic and together with Leu22Pro is causative of disease in individual 373.1.

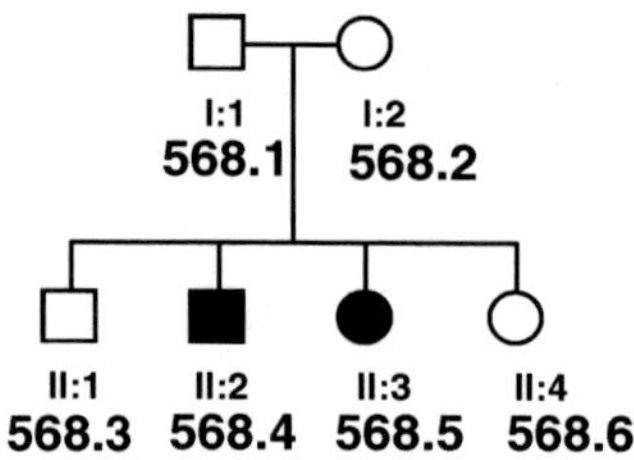

Individual	Mutation	Age of Onset	Visual Acuity	Other clinical information
568.1	Heterozygous IVS1+1G>T	No apparent manifestation		
568.2	Heterozygous Tyr249Cys + Ala132Thr	No apparent manifestation		
568.3	Heterozygous IVS1+1G>T	No apparent manifestation		
568.4	Compound Heterozygote IVS1+1G>T; Tyr249Cys + Ala132Thr	2 months	Age 27: Light perception	
568.5	Compound Heterozygote IVS1+1G>T; Tyr249Cys + Ala132Thr	2 years	Age 25: 6/60 (left eye) 6/120 (right eye)	Photophobia, diffuse RP, waxy pallor of discs, attenuated arteries, bony spicules, markedly thinned retinas, atrophic macula, rapid deterioration of vision from the age of 7, Keratoconus, ERG at age 22 shows advanced rod and cone dysfunction. Vision appeared stable at age 26.
568.6	None			

Figure 1. Pedigree and clinical information of family 568, in which three *RPE65* variants were identified.

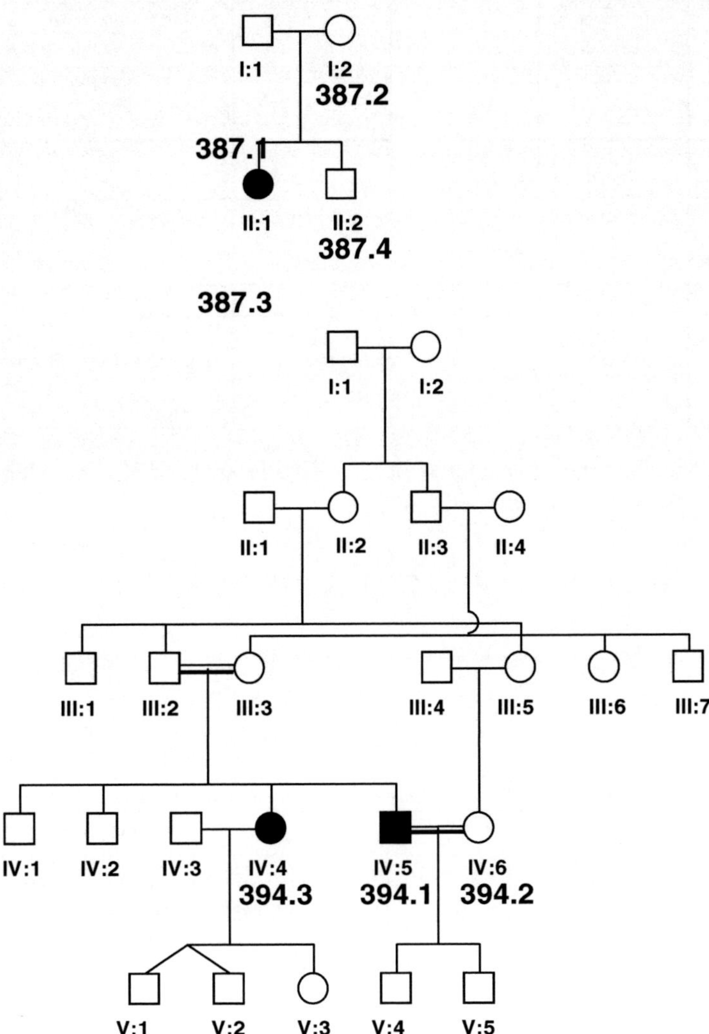

Individual	Mutation	Age of Onset	Visual Acuity	Other clinical information
387.1	Heterozygous Ala132Thr	No apparent manifestation		
387.2	None			

Figure 2. (Continued).

387.3	Heterozygous Ala132Thr	2	Age 4: 6/108 (left eye) 6/36 (right eye) Age 16: 6/60 (both eyes)	Markedly abnormal (flat) ERG at age 2, less than 5° visual field at age 16.
387.4	Heterozygous Ala132Thr	No apparent manifestation		
394.1	Heterozygous Ala132Thr	5	Age 29: 6/120 (left eye) 6/72 (right eye)	Glaucoma at age 29.
394.2	None			
394.3	Heterozygous Ala132Thr	8	Age 32: 6/18 (left eye) 6/70 (right eye)	Diffuse RP, Less than 10° visual fields left at age 32, slow progression in the last 10 years. Cataracts.

Figure 2. Pedigrees and clinical information of families 394 and 387, in which only the Ala132Thr mutation was identified.

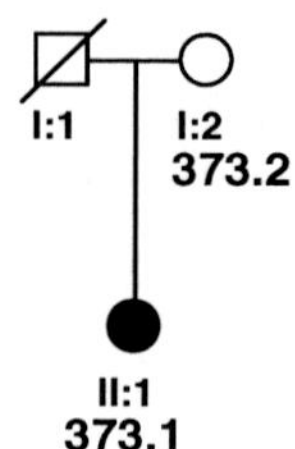

Individual	Mutation	Age of Onset	Visual Acuity	Other clinical information
373.1	Compound Heterozygote Glu21Lys; Leu22Pro	3	Age: 36: 6/15 (left eye) 6/24 (right eye) Age 38: 6/30 (left eye) 6/40 (right eye)	High myopia and nightblindness at age 3, Flat rod and cones ERG response by age 8. Progressive central vision loss at age 37 with typical waxy white discs, attenuated vessels, choroidal atrophy of the right macula, singular bony spicules and significant white punctuate lesions. Cataracts extracted at age 38.
373.2	Heterozygous Glu21Lys	No apparent manifestation		

Figure 3. Pedigree and clinical information of family 373, in which the Glu21Lys and Leu22Pro mutations were identified.

A dHPLC profile variation was observed in exon 10 of one proband with RP. Sequencing of this sample, 52.1, revealed the presence of a homozygous Tyr368His (c.1102T>C) mutation. This variation has been reported as being pathogenic, due to the significant change caused to the protein structure by replacement of a negatively charged tyrosine with a positively charged histidine [31]. This mutation creates an *Alw26 I* restriction enzyme site, so a restriction enzyme digest was performed in order to study the segregation of the mutation in family 52, a Mixed Ancestry family. The mutation was detected in the homozygous state in 52.1, in the heterozygous state in one parent (52.2) and was absent in the stepsibling (52.3). No DNA sample was available from the other parent (Figure 4).

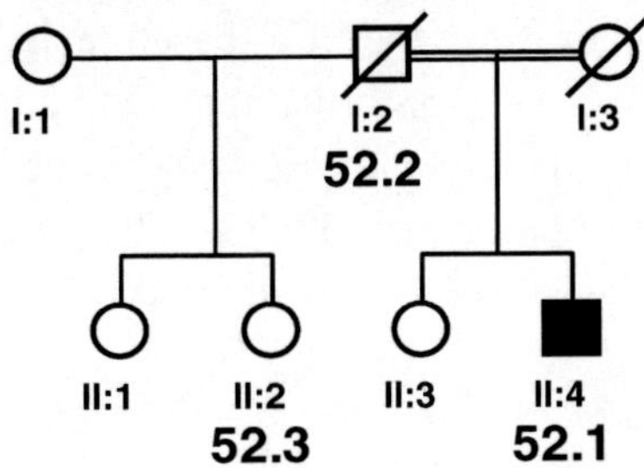

Individual	Mutation	Age of Onset	Visual Acuity	Other clinical information
52.1	Homozygous Tyr368His	4	Age 36: 6/60 (left eye), Counting fingers (right eye)	Early loss of fields, loss of colour vision, RP tigroid fundus, drusen in macula, white dots, waxy pallor, attenuated vessels, choroidal atrophy.
52.2	Heterozygous Tyr368His	No apparent manifestation		
52.3	None			

Figure 4. Pedigree and clinical information of family 52, in which a homozygous Tyr36His mutation was identified.

Conclusion

Five different pathogenic mutations were identified in the 69 individuals with early onset RP (7.3%). This is greater than the reported frequency of 2%

[5], however the current study used an enriched cohort by including only individuals with an age of onset younger than 15 years. No pathogenic mutations in *RPE65* were identified in any of the individuals with LCA, which was unexpected given the reported frequency of 16%.

Five families with RP were found to carry *RPE65* mutations, although the full complement of mutations was identified in only three families while the remaining two families carried the same heterozygous mutation. Sequencing of the entire *RPE65* gene was not performed during the course of this investigation. The second mutation, if it exists in these families, may thus be located in a portion of the gene not analysed in this mutation screening programme, for example the promoter region or deep intronic regions. It should also be considered that large deletions spanning one or more exons would go undetected when using the PCR-based techniques employed in this study. There is the additional possibility that the causative mutation(s) may exist in another gene – whilst digenic effects have not been reported for LCA, modifier effects have been described [32, 33]. The previously reported *RPE65* modifier, Leu450Met, was not detected in this investigation, but recent microarray analysis has revealed that 7% of LCA cases have potential pathogenic variations in more than one gene [32]. This may be the case in the individual with LCA, who was found in this study to carry a heterozygous Asn321Lys variant in *RPE65* and in a subsequent study was found to carry a homozygous Ser175Arg mutation in the *LRAT* gene. It is possible that the *RPE65* variant may be a modifier of the disease phenotype caused by the *LRAT* mutations. It is also possible that the third variant (Tyr249Cys) identified in a family with two pathogenic mutations (IVS1+1G>T and Ala132Thr) may modify disease in these individuals. Functional analysis should be performed to ascertain the disease relevance of the novel Tyr249Cys sequence variation.

The Ala132Thr mutation was the single most common variation detected, as it was identified in three of the 69 individuals classified as having RP (4.4%). Interestingly, two of these three individuals were of Indian descent. In light of the fact that the immigrant populations contributing to the rich ethnic and cultural diversity in SA include those from southern India, northern India and Pakistan [34], the Ala132Thr mutation may represent a mutation seen in the east. However, to the best of our knowledge this has not been reported. It is also interesting that the 'Dutch founder Tyr368His mutation' was not more prevalent in the SA cohort (a reasonable fraction of whom would be of Dutch descent) and that this mutation was only identified in the homozygous state in a family of Mixed Ancestry. The haplotype surrounding the Tyr368His mutation in this Mixed Ancestry family was not compared to that of the original Dutch families, and this may be considered for future research.

The full mutation complement was identified in three families in this SA cohort. Molecular genetic results which have arisen from RDD research are delivered to patients according to a previously described protocol [35], which was established by a management team that included medical geneticists, genetic counsellors, medical scientists and a clinical coordinator. Following result delivery to one patient, she wrote a letter to the lay support group Retina South Africa which was published in the newsletter Retina E-News no 5, January 2008:

Excerpt from "A Letter of Hope"

I am a 28 year old female advocate and I am partially sighted.

I received a call from my branch secretary, advising me that I should attend a genetic counselling session at the national office of Retina South Africa in order to obtain the results of my gene tracking. I agreed, however with no real zest. My view was that I would probably receive the result and that would be it. HOWEVER to my astonishment I was overwhelmed to find out that the gene affected is RPE65, YES which means that I was at the right place at the right time, given the fact that clinical trials have already begun on this specific gene type.

I must admit it took a while for this newly found info to register, however when it really sunk in, and I realized what all of this meant, I uncontrollably burst into tears of happiness. Not only has the root of the problem been found, but there is also HOPE that accompanies it…

A lesson well learnt: Never give up, because there is always hope and light at the end of the tunnel.

In light of the fact that the efficacy of *RPE65* gene replacement therapy may be improved if applied in children, it would be worthwhile to consider screening of schools for the visually impaired in order to identify children with arRP and LCA in SA. However, given that no *RPE65* mutations were identified in the LCA cohort in this study, future mutation screening should be performed using microarray technology rather than the traditional, laborious whole-gene analysis methods. It would appear that the most prevalent genetic defects which cause RDD in other parts of the world are present in SA patient cohorts at an almost insignificant incidence [36-39]. The use of microarrays will enable the screening of multiple genes simultaneously, which may lead to the characterisation of the unique SA RDD molecular profile and in turn allow patients to benefit from gene therapy intervention, such as that of the *RPE65* version of LCA.

Acknowledgements

We are indebted to all families with inherited retinal degenerative disorders in South Africa for their participation in this research program. We are grateful to Daneel Lambrechts who performed some of the mutation analysis. We thank Sister Lecia Bartmann and Ms. Ncumisa Zitho, the clinical coordinators on the RDD program. This study was funded by Retina South Africa, the University of Cape Town, the South African Medical Research Council, and the Technology and Human Resources for Industry Programme of the National Research Fund (South Africa).

References

[1]   Nicoletti, A; Wong, DJ; Kawase, K; Gibson, LH; Yang-Feng, TL; Richards, JE; Thompson, DA. Molecular characterization of the human gene encoding an abundant 61 kDa protein specific to the retinal pigment epithelium. *Hum Mol Genet.*, 1995, 4(4), 641-649.

[2]   Moiseyev, G; Chen, Y; Takahashi, Y; Wu, BX; Ma, JX. RPE65 is the isomerohydrolase in the retinoid visual cycle. *Proc Natl Acad Sci.*, USA, 2005, 102(35), 12413-12418.

[3]   Redmond, TM; Yu, S; Lee, E; Bok, D; Hamasaki, D; Chen, N; Goletz, P; Ma, JX; Crouch, RK; Pfeifer, K. Rpe65 is necessary for production of 11-cis-vitamin A in the retinal visual cycle. *Nat Genet.*, 1998, 20(4), 344-351.

[4]   Pang, JJ; Chang, B; Hawes, NL; Hurd, RE; Davisson, MT; Li, J; Noorwez, SM; Malhotra, R; McDowell, JH; Kaushal, S; Hauswirth, WW; Nusinowitz, S; Thompson, DA; Heckenlively, JR. Retinal

degeneration 12 (rd12): a new, spontaneously arising mouse model for human Leber congenital amaurosis (LCA). *Mol Vis.*, 2005, 11, 152-162.

[5]   Morimura, H; Fishman, GA; Grover, SA; Fulton, AB; Berson, EL; Dryja, TP. Mutations in the RPE65 gene in patients with autosomal recessive retinitis pigmentosa or leber congenital amaurosis. *Proc Natl Acad Sci.*, U S A., 1998, 95(6), 3088-3093.

[6]   Cremers, FP; van den Hurk, JA; den Hollander, AI. Molecular genetics of Leber congenital amaurosis. *Hum Mol Genet.*, 2002, 11(10), 1169-1176.

[7]   Hims, MM; Diager, SP; Inglehearn, CF. Retinitis pigmentosa: genes, proteins and prospects. *Dev Ophthalmol.*, 2003, 37, 109-125.

[8]   Wenzel, A; Reme, CE; Williams, TP; Hafezi, F; Grimm, C. The Rpe65 Leu450Met variation increases retinal resistance against light-induced degeneration by slowing rhodopsin regeneration. *J Neurosci.*, 2001, 21(1), 53-58.

[9]   Samardzija, M; Wenzel, A; Naash, M; Reme, CE; Grimm, C. Rpe65 as a modifier gene for inherited retinal degeneration. *Eur J Neurosci.*, 2006, 23(4), 1028-1034.

[10]   Wenzel, A; Grimm, C; Samardzija, M; Reme, CE. The genetic modifier Rpe65Leu(450): effect on light damage susceptibility in c-Fos-deficient mice. *Invest Ophthalmol Vis Sci.*, 2003, 44(6), 2798-2802.

[11]   Acland, GM; Aguirre, GD; Ray, J; Zhang, Q; Aleman, TS; Cideciyan, AV; Pearce-Kelling, SE; Anand, V; Zeng, Y; Maguire, AM; Jacobson, SG; Hauswirth, WW; Bennett, J. Gene therapy restores vision in a canine model of childhood blindness. *Nat Genet.*, 2001 28(1), 92-95.

[12]   Acland, GM; Aguirre, GD; Bennett, J; Aleman, TS; Cideciyan, AV; Bennicelli, J; Dejneka, NS; Pearce-Kelling, SE; Maguire, AM; Palczewski, K; Hauswirth, WW; Jacobson, SG. Long-term restoration of rod and cone vision by single dose rAAV-mediated gene transfer to the retina in a canine model of childhood blindness. *Mol Ther.*, 2005, 12(6), 1072-1082.

[13]   Pang, JJ; Chang, B; Kumar, A; Nusinowitz, S; Noorwez, SM; Li, J; Rani, A; Foster, TC; Chiodo, VA; Doyle, T; Li, H; Malhotra, R; Teusner, JT; McDowell, JH; Min, SH; Li, Q; Kaushal, S; Hauswirth, WW. Gene therapy restores vision-dependent behavior as well as retinal structure and function in a mouse model of RPE65 Leber congenital amaurosis. *Mol Ther.*, 2006, 13(3), 565-572.

[14] Chen, Y; Moiseyev, G; Takahashi, Y; Ma, JX. RPE65 gene delivery restores isomerohydrolase activity and prevents early cone loss in Rpe65-/- mice. *Invest Ophthalmol Vis Sci.*, 2006, 47(3), 1177-1184.

[15] Hauswirth, WW. The consortium project to treat RPE65 deficiency in humans. *Retina.*, 2005, 25(8 Suppl), S60.

[16] Bainbridge, JW; Smith, AJ; Barker, SS; Robbie, S; Henderson, R; Balaggan, K; Viswanathan, A; Holder, GE; Stockman, A; Tyler, N; Petersen-Jones, S; Bhattacharya, SS; Thrasher, AJ; Fitzke, FW; Carter, BJ; Rubin, GS; Moore, AT; Ali, RR. Effect of gene therapy on visual function in Leber's congenital amaurosis. *N Engl J Med.*, 2008, 358(21), 2231-2239.

[17] Maguire, AM; Simonelli, F; Pierce, EA; Pugh, EN Jr.; Mingozzi, F; Bennicelli, J; Banfi, S; Marshall, KA; Testa, F; Surace, EM; Rossi, S; Lyubarsky, A; Arruda, VR; Konkle, B; Stone, E; Sun, J; Jacobs, J; Dell'Osso, L; Hertle, R; Ma, JX; Redmond, TM; Zhu, X; Hauck, B; Zelenaia, O; Shindler, KS; Maguire, MG; Wright, JF; Volpe, NJ; McDonnell, JW; Auricchio, A; High, KA; Bennett, J. Safety and efficacy of gene transfer for Leber's congenital amaurosis. *N Engl J Med.*, 2008, 358(21), 2240-2248.

[18] Hauswirth, WW; Aleman, TS; Kaushal, S; Cideciyan, AV; Schwartz, SB; Wang, L; Conlon, TJ; Boye, SL; Flotte, TR; Byrne, BJ; Jacobson, SG. Treatment of leber congenital amaurosis due to RPE65 mutations by ocular subretinal injection of adeno-associated virus gene vector: short-term results of a phase I trial. *Hum Gene Ther.*, 2008, 19(10), 979-990.

[19] Botha, MC; Beighton, P. Inherited disorders in the Afrikaner population of southern Africa. Part I. Historical and demographic background, cardiovascular, neurological, metabolic and intestinal conditions. *S Afr Med J.*, 1983, 64(16), 609-612.

[20] Groenewald, JZ; Liebenberg, J; Groenewald, IM; Warnich, L. Linkage disequilibrium analysis in a recently founded population: evaluation of the variegate porphyria founder in South African Afrikaners. *Am J Hum Genet.*, 1998, 62(5), 1254-1258.

[21] Defesche, JC; van Diermen, DE; Lansberg, PJ; Lamping, RJ; Reymer, PW; Hayden, MR; Kastelein, JJ. South African founder mutations in the low-density lipoprotein receptor gene causing familial hyper-cholesterolemia in the Dutch population. *Hum Genet.*, 1993, 92(6), 567-570.

[22] Yzer, S; van den Born, LI; Schuil, J; Kroes, HY; van Genderen, MM; Boonstra, FN; van den Helm, B; Brunner, HG; Koenekoop, RK; Cremers, FP. A Tyr368His RPE65 founder mutation is associated with variable expression and progression of early onset retinal dystrophy in 10 families of a genetically isolated population. *J Med Genet.*, 2003, 40(9), 709-713.

[23] Greenberg, J; Bartmann, L; Ramesar, R; Beighton, P. Retinitis pigmentosa in southern Africa. *Clin Genet.*, 1993, 44(5), 232-235.

[24] Ramesar, RS; Roberts, L; Rebello, G; Goliath, R; Vorster, A; September, A; Ehrenreich, L; Gama, D; Greenberg, J. Retinal degenerative disorders in Southern Africa: a molecular genetic approach. *Adv Exp Med Biol.*, 2003, 533, 35-40.

[25] Cotton, RG; Scriver, CR. Proof of "disease causing" mutation. *Hum Mutat.*, 1998, 12(1), 1-3.

[26] Reese, MG; Eeckmann, FH. Splice Sites: A detailed neural network study. In: *Genome Mapping & Sequencing Meeting*; 1996, Cold Spring Harbour, New York; 1996.

[27] Reese, MG; Eeckman, FH; Kulp, D; Haussler, D. Improved splice site detection in Genie. *J Comput Biol.*, 1997, 4(3), 311-323.

[28] Thompson, DA; Gyurus, P; Fleischer, LL; Bingham, EL; McHenry, CL; Apfelstedt-Sylla, E; Zrenner, E; Lorenz, B; Richards, JE; Jacobson, SG; Sieving, PA; Gal, A. Genetics and phenotypes of RPE65 mutations in inherited retinal degeneration. *Invest Ophthalmol Vis Sci.*, 2000, 41(13), 4293-4299.

[29] Philpa, AR; Jin, M; Li, S; Schindler, EI; Iannaccone, A; Lam, BL; Weleber, RG; Fishman, GA; Jacobson, SG; Mullins, RF; Travis, GH; Stone, EM. Predicting the pathogenicity of RPE65 mutations. *Hum Mutat.*, 2009, 30(5), 1-6.

[30] Marlhens, F; Griffoin, JM; Bareil, C; Arnaud, B; Claustres, M; Hamel, CP. Autosomal recessive retinal dystrophy associated with two novel mutations in the RPE65 gene. *Eur J Hum Genet.*, 1998, 6(5), 527-531.

[31] Lorenz, B; Gyurus, P; Preising, M; Bremser, D; Gu, S; Andrassi, M; Gerth, C; Gal, A. Early-onset severe rod-cone dystrophy in young children with RPE65 mutations. *Invest Ophthalmol Vis Sci.*, 2000, 41(9), 2735-2742.

[32] Zernant, J; Kulm, M; Dharmaraj, S; den Hollander, AI; Perrault, I; Preising, MN; Lorenz, B; Kaplan, J; Cremers, FP; Maumenee, I; Koenekoop, RK; Allikmets, R. Genotyping microarray (disease chip) for

Leber congenital amaurosis: detection of modifier alleles. *Invest Ophthalmol Vis Sci.*, 2005, 46(9), 3052-3059.

[33] Silva, E; Dharmaraj, S; Li, YY; Pina, AL; Carter, RC; Loyer, M; Traboulsi, E; Theodossiadis, G; Koenekoop, R; Sundin, O; Maumenee, I. A missense mutation in GUCY2D acts as a genetic modifier in RPE65-related Leber Congenital Amaurosis. *Ophthalmic Genet.*, 2004, 25(3), 205-217.

[34] Beighton, P; Sellars, SL; Goldblatt, J; Viljoen, DL; Beighton, G. Childhood deafness in the Indian population of Natal. *S Afr Med J.*, 1987, 72(3), 209-211.

[35] Roberts, L; Rebello, G; Ramesar, R; Greenberg, J. Management of a South African family with retinitis pigmentosa - should potential therapy influence translational research protocols? *J ocul biol dis inform.*, 2008, 1, 55-58.

[36] Greenberg, J; Roberts, L; Ramesar, R. Unusual frequencies of Rhodopsin mutations and polymorphisms in South African patients with Retinitis Pigmentosa. In: R. E. Anderson, M.M. LaVail & J. G. Hollyfield (Eds.), *New insights into retinal degenerative diseases.* Proceedings of the 9th International Symposium on Retinal Degeneration; 2000 2001; Durango, CO: Kluwer Academic/Plenum Publishers; 2000, 329-333.

[37] Roberts, L; Ramesar, R; Greenberg, J. Low frequency of rhodopsin mutations in South African patients with autosomal dominant retinitis pigmentosa. *Clin Genet.*, 2000, 58(1), 77-78.

[38] Roberts, L; Bartmann, L; Ramesar, R; Greenberg, J. Novel variants in the hotspot region of RP1 in South African patients with retinitis pigmentosa. *Mol Vis.*, 2006, 12, 177-183.

[39] September, AV; Vorster, AA; Ramesar, RS; Greenberg, LJ. Mutation spectrum and founder chromosomes for the ABCA4 gene in South African patients with Stargardt disease. *Invest Ophthalmol Vis Sci.*, 2004 45(6), 1705-1711.

In: Reginitis Pigmentosa: Causes, Diagnosis…   ISBN: 978-1-60876-884-4
Editors: M. Baert, et al. pp. 111-125   © 2010 Nova Science Publishers, Inc.

Chapter IV

Diagnosis and Treatment of Retinitis Pigmentosa Based on the Pathology

Catherine Cukras[*] and Chi-Chao Chan
National Eye Institute, National Institutes of Health, Bethesda, MD, USA.

Abstract

Retinitis pigmentosa (RP) is a group of inherited retinal degenerations, caused by mutations in one of many genes - some already identified, and some still yet to be discovered. While there are many different genes involved and great heterogeneity among these genes, the underlying common source of vision loss is retinal dysfunction related to photoreceptor loss. The sequence of histopathologic changes associated with RP occurs in several stages. The 1st stage is associated with rod photoreceptor dysfunction and ultimate death and the second with cone photoreceptor demise. Following photoreceptor loss, a number of secondary changes occur, with retinal pigment epithelial (RPE) cells detaching from of Bruch's membrane and migrating into the inner retina to ultimately accumulate and surround blood vessels which gives rise to the "bone spicules" observed clinically. Other pathologies include

---

[*] Corresponding author: E-mail: cukrasc@nei.nih.gov

attenuation of blood vessels, retinal gliosis, migration of microglia into the outer retina, optic nerve atrophy and mild vitritis. Current therapies for RP include: genetic replacement of missing/mutated proteins via viral vectors, addition (by injection or surgery) of factors or supplements that may prolong photoreceptor survival, transplantation of photoreceptors and RPE cells and electrical stimulation of remaining neurons, as well as developing therapies targeted at preventing photoreceptor apoptosis. Understanding the histopathologic changes occurring in RP is critical to understanding the rationale for current therapies, as well as to develop future therapies. Mouse models of retinitis pigmentosa, have been instrumental in aiding the study of histopathologic changes that occur in the setting of retinitis pigmentosa and to initiate and study various treatment approaches. Many of the findings of the histopathologic changes and treatment avenues are explored in these models.

Introduction

Retinitis pigmentosa (RP) is a group of inherited retinal degenerations, caused by mutations in one of many genes - some already identified, and some still yet to be discovered. Dr. Donders first described the disease in 1857.[1] The name itself is derived from the clinical and pathologic findings. The term "retinitis" refers to inflammation in the form of a mild vitritis, and "pigmentosa" refers to the pigmentation that accumulates as "bone spicules" around the retinal vasculature in the periphery. While there are many different genes involved and great heterogeneity among these genes, the underlying common source of vision loss is retinal dysfunction related to photoreceptor loss. Following photoreceptor loss, several pathological changes have been documented to occur to ultimately give the clinical picture characteristic of RP.

Knowledge of the histopathologic changes that occur in RP is critical to understanding the rationale for current therapies, as well as developing future therapies. Mouse models of retinitis pigmentosa have been instrumental in aiding the study of histopathologic changes that occur in the setting of RP and to initiate and investigate various treatment approaches. Many of the findings of the histopathologic features and treatment avenues are explored in these models.

Histological Features in RP

The sequence of histopathologic changes associated with RP occurs in several stages, which provides insight into potential targets for therapy. The initial stage is associated with rod photoreceptor dysfunction and ultimate death followed by cone photoreceptor demise. In advanced cases, most photoreceptors are absent and the remaining few are in the periphery near the ora serrata.[2]

Different genetic mutations cause different proteins to be affected in different ways – some mutations lead to the incorrect trafficking of the protein, whereas others lead to the proper localization of the protein, but cause problems with phototransduction itself or photoreceptor-RPE interactions.[3-5] Regardless of the genetic mutation, the the shorting of rod photoreceptor outer segments is the initial pathologic change seen in genetic RP is.[2, 6] The mid-peripheral or equatorial retina is typically the first location where the rod outer segment shortening occurs.[7] Progression of rod photoreceptor loss then projects both inwards toward the macula and outwards toward the retinal periphery. The mechanism whereby mutations in a given protein result in the death of rod photoreceptors is unknown in most cases.[8] The process ultimately is thought to involve caspases in apoptosis[9-12] although some recent evidence indicates that there also may be non-caspase dependent mechanisms, such as necrosis-like programmed cell death or autophagy, responsible for photoreceptor cell death.[13] It is this loss or atrophy of rod photoreceptors that produces the first clinical symptoms of night vision difficulties, or nyctalopia in RP.

Following extensive rod photoreceptor loss, cones, too, are lost universally in RP, regardless of genetic form. Clinically, this is observed in the electroretinogram (ERG) responses which show rod-derived responses affected earlier, and to a greater degree, than cone-derived responses.[14] Interestingly, cone degeneration even occurs in forms of RP where the mutant protein is not expressed in cones. The mechanism by which the mutated RP protein ultimately leads to cone demise is not completely understood but has led to two main hypotheses: 1) cone degeneration results from a lack of trophic factors normally produced from functioning rods;[15-17] or 2) cone cell death is caused by the release of toxic byproducts or other activated processes initiated by degenerating rod photoreceptors.[4, 18] It is this secondary loss of cone cells that is responsible for much of the vision loss in these patients. In advanced RP, the macula may show a loss of all rod cells and most cones, but typically, remaining cones can be seen histologically as a monolayer of cone somata with shortened outer segments.[2, 9]

Secondary Changes

Following photoreceptor loss, a number of secondary changes occur. Retinal pigment epithelial (RPE) cells detach from Bruch's membrane and migrate into the inner retina. RPE cells ultimately accumulate and surround blood vessels which gives rise to the "bone spicules" observed clinically[9] (Figure 1 and 2). The inciting factors for RPE migration remain unknown, but are thought to be secondary to the loss of photoreceptors disrupting the interdependent relationship of these two cells. Also, the reasoning for relocation of RPE cells to the perivascular region is not known, but has been hypothesized to stem from an affinity of RPE cells for the vascular basal laminae.[9]

There are many repercussions from the migration of RPE cells. The loss of RPE cells, combined with the demise of photoreceptors and extension of **Muller cells towards Bruch's membrane, leads to a loss of the subretinal** space.[7] Further, as RPE cells encircle the vasculature several changes occur. Deposits laid down in the extracellular matrix by migrated RPE cells have been noted to resemble the five-**layered structure of Bruch's membrane**[8] and are often so thick as to physically compress the vasculature.[7] Clinically, this is observed as the attenuation and narrowing of retina vessels. In some cases, the vessels actually become occluded.[7] Vascular change is thought to contribute to the degeneration of the inner retina seen in late stages of RP.[8] RPE cell migration to the small retinal vessels also leads to a change in the function of the vascular endothelium. This is observed histologically as an increase in fenestrations in the vessels which are encircled by RPE cells[9] and observed clinically as leakage on fluorescein angiography.

The choriocapillaris also has a close interdependence on both the RPE and photoreceptors and becomes atrophic soon after the migration of the RPE. The atrophy of the choriocapillaris does not appear to be specific to RP, but, rather has been noted to follow the loss of RPE in several pathological conditions.[19]

Muller cells also undergo activation and retinal gliosis (proliferation of retinal glial cells) as a non-specific reaction in RP, among other degenerations.[20] This reactive gliosis can be observed histopathologically in advanced RP as hypertrophied Muller cells and hyperplastic glial cells strongly reactive for glial fibrillary acidic protein (GFAP)[9] with thickened cell processes in the space of the degenerated photoreceptors.[7] It is also evidenced in their presence in the epiretinal membranes (ERMs) [21] that afflict more than 80% of patients with RP (Figure 3). The activation and migration of microglia has been noted to occur in RP and also in other retinal degenerations following the loss of rod photoreceptors where they phagocytose photoreceptor debris.[22, 23] In histologic sections of human retinas with RP[9] and AMD[24] the presence of microglia in the outer retina has been found to follow photoreceptor atrophy. Additionally, mild inflammatory cells, particularly macrophages, have been found in the vitreous and retina.

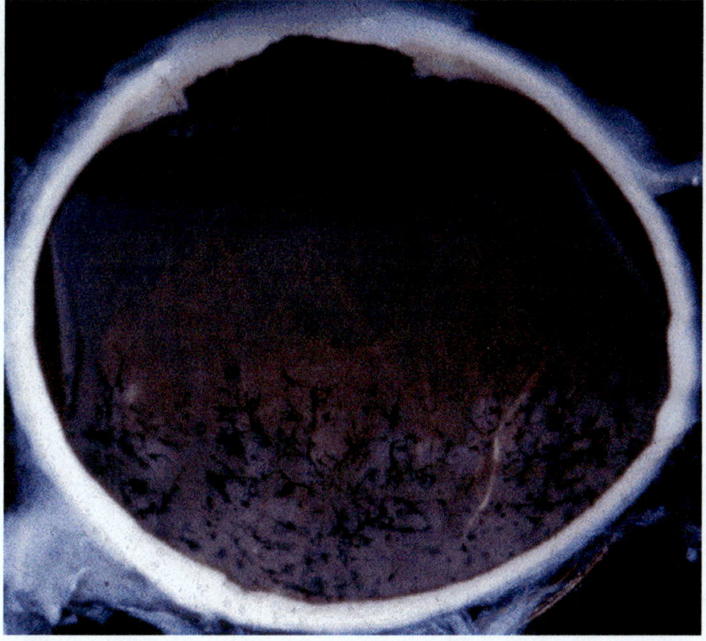

Figure 1. Gross pathology of an eye with Retinitis Pigmentosa showing pigmentary accumulation in, a "bone spicule" pattern.

Treatments

Current therapies for RP span a wide spectrum of strategies and treatment modalities ranging from vitamin supplementation to genetic replacement of missing/mutated proteins to developing therapies targeted at preventing photoreceptor apoptosis. Close attention to the histologic characteristics of RP afflicted eyes will provide insight into the potential hurdles of various treatment approaches.

Vitamin Supplementation

As a consequence of the loss of rod cells, the milleu of the interphotoreceptor matrix (IPM) is significantly changed.[25] Since proteins involved in the visual cycle are affected, the local environment of the cells is altered potentially leading to a type of local vitamin A deficiency in cones.[7] Clinical evidence to support this hypothesis are the results of Berson et al, which has shown that supplementation of vitamin A in people with RP slowed cone degeneration, as evidenced by changes in the ERG.[26]

Gene Therapy

The molecular basis for photoreceptor dysfunction is known in a large number of cases and is caused by various mutations in several different genes. To date, over 40 genes have been identified causing clinical RP (Retnet database, www.sph.uth.tmc.edu/retnet, information retrieved in June 2009). Some of the proteins affected are unique to the retina, and thus cause a purely retinal phenotype, whereas others are also expressed in additional tissues and comprise one of the 30 known RP syndromes.[7] Gene therapy is attractive for genetic diseases, but seems daunting due to the number of mutations involved in clinical RP. The protein products of the involved genes span structural proteins, such as myosin VIIA involved in RPE and photoreceptor cells in Usher syndrome type 1B,[27, 28] to proteins involved directly in phototransduction such as rhodopsin and alpha and beta phosphodiesterase.[29, 30]

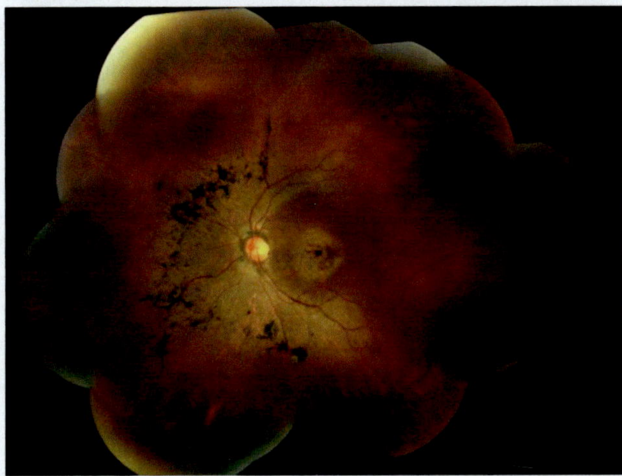

Figure 2. Montage of fundus photographs of an eye with advanced retinitis pigmentosa showing pigmentary changes in the mid-periphery and an abnormal macula..

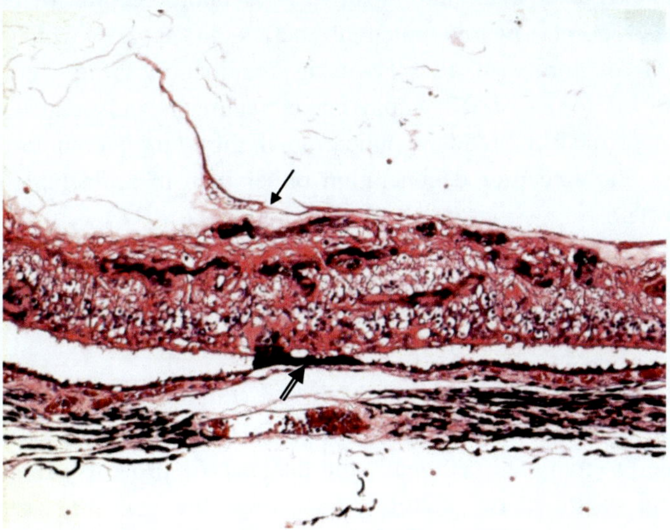

Figure 3: Histologic section including the neurosensory retina and choroid of an eye with retinitis pigmentosa. Note the presence of an epiretinal membrane (arrow) seen as a thin fibrotic sheet of cells at the retina/vitreous interface. The retina shows a total loss of photoreceptor cells and RPE migration into the retina and surrounding sclerotic retinal vessels. There is chorioretinal scar with RPE hypertrophy (double line arrow). Few inflammatory cells are seen in the vitreous. (hematoxylin & eosin, original magnifiction, x100)

Another hurdle facing gene therapy is the mode of delivering the gene. Gene therapy approaches in animal models, and in human trials thus far, have mostly involved delivery of a viral vector to the subretinal space.[31-34] As noted above, the architecture of the subretinal space in RP patients is significantly altered, with substantial loss of this potential space. The development of alternative methods of gene delivery may hold promise and new delivery systems are currently being investigated. For example, liposome and polymer-mediated delivery systems are non-viral systems which involve subretinal injections for delivery to the photoreceptors.[35] Intravitreal injection of viral vectors[36] is potentially attractive as it would circumvent the difficulties incurred by the histologic changes observed in the subretinal space in these patients.

Despite the variety of genetic mutations involved, there are common histopathological findings between the various genetic mutations in RP, particularly in the late stage, which indicate that the disease follows the same course and suggests a common pathway of photoreceptor demise. These findings also point towards potential therapeutic targets which might be common to all forms of RP. Focusing therapeutic targets on pathways common to all forms of RP would make treatments universal. Gene-based therapies may have a broader application if they target common pathways involved in photoreceptor degeneration rather than in replacing the specific mutated protein.

Targeting Apoptosis

Apoptosis, or programmed cell-death, is a common pathway thought to be involved in the ultimate demise of photoreceptors.[37] The exact mechanism of apoptotic programmed cell death and the specific proteins involved is still controversial with some results supporting the role of caspases in photoreceptor apoptosis,[38, 39] while others suggest that the death of photoreceptors may be secondary to caspase-independent mechanisms.[40, 41] Studies show that while caspase-dependent mechanisms may be important in apoptosis involved in development, they are downregulated in post-mitotic cells. The reports of the effects of caspase inhibitors are variable and, in some studies, have been shown to have only a transient effect in animal models of retinal degeneration.[39] Caspase-independent mechanisms, such as calpains, granzymes and cathepsins, have been proposed to be involved in stress-related apoptosis.[42] In particular, calcium and calpains have been shown to be key players in animal models of retinal degenerations.[43]

The hypothesis that calcium may play an important role in photoreceptor death has led to the investigation of various calcium channel blockers in the treatment of mouse models RP.[38] From microarray analysis, investigators were able to analyze the genes affected by the inhibition of calcium channels. It was shown that altering calcium levels had many effects including altering the expression of calcium binding proteins important in metabolism, in apoptosis, and in synaptic function.[38, 44]

Trophic Factors

Several diffusible factors have been identified which promote photoreceptor survival. Basic fibroblast growth factor (bFGF) is one such factor which has been shown to induce photoreceptor survival in animal models of retina degeneration.[15, 45, 46] Other factors identified include: Leukemia Inhibitory factor (LIF), which has been shown to be able to protect photoreceptor cells against light-induced photoreceptor degeneration;[47] rod-derived cone viability factor (RdCVF), which is believed to increase cone survival;[48] glial cell-derived neurotrophic factor (GDNF);[49] and ciliary neurotrophic factor.[50] Administration of these factors, which are believed to be neuroprotective, has been accomplished both by subretinal delivery and by intravitreal administration.[46, 51] As per the discussion above describing changes to the subretinal space in RP, delivery via an intravitreal route would have advantages over subretinal delivery, due to a distortion and loss of this potential space in diseased retinas. Methods of delivery of these proteins include direct injection of the protein into the vitreous[48] and encapsulation of modified cells,[50] which attempts to harness the protein secreting capabilities of these cells.[49, 52]

Beyond the technical and surgical considerations, it is likely that these factors that help support the survival of photoreceptors will be potential therapies only in the earlier phases of the disease. For the case where photoreceptor demise has already occurred, and when RPE has already affected and migrated, it is likely that these treatment options will not be sufficient to address the pathology.

Role of microglia

Microglia in the central nervous system have been found to produce nitrous oxide and other cytotoxic products, which are involved in the death of neurons. By extension, microglia activation and migration in the retina is thought to be associated with the release of cytotoxic factors and the death of photoreceptors.[53] However, the precise role of microglia in the pathogenesis of RP is still debated. Targeting microglia with various inhibitors appears to be promising in mouse models of retinal degeneration. For example, naloxone has been shown to prolong photoreceptor survival in the light-induced retinal degeneration animal model[54]. Furhter, minocycline, another microglia inhibitor, has been shown to delay photoreceptor death in the rds mouse. However, others have found that bone-marrow activation of microglia can actually lead to a deceleration of retinal degeneration and the survival of cones.[55] Further investigation of the role of microglia likely will lead to better targeted therapies.

Cell transplantation

Histology reveals that RP is not only a photoreceptor disease but that RPE cells are lost as well, along with the eventual atrophy of the choriocapillaris. Replacing photoreceptors, which is still in preliminary phases, must take into account the anatomic changes that will likely make this approach more difficult. The loss of the subretinal space by both RPE migration and, therefore, chorioretinal adhesion or scarring in this space, and the extensive gliosis **to Bruch's membrane makes this surgically more challenging. In cases** where the RPE has already migrated through the retina, RPE cells would have to be transplanted, along with the photoceptors.[7] Further, the fenestrations **and "leakiness" of the retinal vasculature** give more concern for potential immune response to the foreign tissue.[8] Some forays into this mode of tissue delivery have been made with transplantation of fetal retina to areas of retinal atrophy in RP patients[56, 57] with relatively good tolerance for the transplanted tissue and the surgery, but further study is needed.

Summary

There are many novel approaches and new techniques being developed in the effort to conquer the challenges of treating RP and there are likely many more emerging as this is written. The information obtained from molecular mechanisms and cellular pathways involved will drive this research, in conjunction with the changes occurring on a cellular level as observed by careful understanding of the histopathology. As others have pointed out, [7, 8] consideration of the entirety of retinal changes – from the protein changes incurred to the restructuring of the retinal architecture – will be critical in the formulation and implementation of treatment strategies.

Bibliography

[1]   Donders, F. Beitrage zur pathologishen Anatomie des Auges. 2. Pigmentbildung in der Netzhaut. *Arch Ophthalmol.*, 1857, 3, 139-165.

[2]   Milam, AH; Li, ZY; Cideciyan, AV; Jacobson, SG. Clinicopathologic effects of the Q64ter rhodopsin mutation in retinitis pigmentosa. *Invest Ophthalmol Vis Sci.*, 1996, 37(5), 753-765.

[3]   Li, T; Snyder, WK; Olsson, JE; Dryja, TP. Transgenic mice carrying the dominant rhodopsin mutation P347S: evidence for defective vectorial transport of rhodopsin to the outer segments. *Proc Natl Acad Sci.*, USA., 1996, 93(24), 14176-14181.

[4]   Bird, AC. Investigation of disease mechanisms in retinitis pigmentosa. *Ophthalmic Paediatr Genet*, 1992, 13(2), 57-66.

[5]   Berson, EL. Retinitis pigmentosa: unfolding its mystery. *Proc Natl Acad Sci.*, U S A., 1996, 93(10), 4526-4528.

[6]   Li, ZY; Jacobson, SG; Milam, AH. Autosomal dominant retinitis pigmentosa caused by the threonine-17-methionine rhodopsin mutation: retinal histopathology and immunocytochemistry. *Exp Eye Res.*, 1994, 58(4), 397-408.

[7]   Milam, AH; Li, ZY; Fariss, RN. Histopathology of the human retina in retinitis pigmentosa. *Prog Retin Eye Res.*, 1998, 17(2), 175-205.

[8]   Milam, AH; Li, ZY. Retinal Pathology in Retinitis Pigmentosa, Considerations for Therapy. In: R. E. Anderson, M. M. LaVail, & J. G.

Hollyfield (Eds.), *Degenerative Diseases of the Retina*. Plenum Press: New York, 1995, 275-284.

[9] Li, ZY; Possin, DE; Milam, AH. Histopathology of bone spicule pigmentation in retinitis pigmentosa. *Ophthalmology*, 1995, 102(5), 805-816.

[10] Chang, GQ; Hao, Y; Wong, F. Apoptosis: final common pathway of photoreceptor death in rd, rds, and rhodopsin mutant mice. *Neuron.*, 1993, 11(4), 595-605.

[11] Adamian, M; Pawlyk, BS; Hong, DH; Berson, EL. Rod and cone opsin mislocalization in an autopsy eye from a carrier of X-linked retinitis pigmentosa with a Gly436Asp mutation in the RPGR gene. *Am J Ophthalmol.*, 2006, 142(3), 515-518.

[12] Lohr, HR; Kuntchithapautham, K; Sharma, AK; Rohrer, B. Multiple, parallel cellular suicide mechanisms participate in photoreceptor cell death. *Exp Eye Res.*, 2006, 83(2), 380-389.

[13] Sancho-Pelluz, J; Arango-Gonzalez, B; Kustermann, S; et al. Photoreceptor cell death mechanisms in inherited retinal degeneration. *Mol Neurobiol.*, 2008, 38(3), 253-269.

[14] Berson, EL. Retinitis pigmentosa. The Friedenwald Lecture. *Invest Ophthalmol Vis Sci.*, 1993, 34(5), 1659-1676.

[15] Steinberg, RH. Survival factors in retinal degenerations. *Curr Opin Neurobiol.*, 1994, 4(4), 515-524.

[16] Mohand-Said, S; Hicks, D; Dreyfus, H; Sahel, JA. Selective transplantation of rods delays cone loss in a retinitis pigmentosa model. *Arch Ophthalmol.*, 2000, 118(6), 807-811.

[17] Milam, AH. Strategies for rescue of retinal photoreceptor cells. *Curr Opin Neurobiol.*, 1993, 3(5), 797-804.

[18] Komeima, K; Rogers, BS; Lu, L; Campochiaro, PA. Antioxidants reduce cone cell death in a model of retinitis pigmentosa. *Proc Natl Acad Sci.*, U S A., 2006, 103(30), 11300-11305.

[19] Korte, GE; Reppucci, V; Henkind, P. RPE destruction causes choriocapillary atrophy. *Invest Ophthalmol Vis Sci.*, 1984, 25(10), 1135-1145.

[20] Henkind, P; Gartner, S. The relationship between retinal pigment epithelium and the choriocapillaris. *Trans Ophthalmol Soc.*, U K., 1983, 103(Pt 4), 444-447.

[21] Szamier, RB. Ultrastructure of the preretinal membrane in retinitis pigmentosa. *Invest Ophthalmol Vis Sci.*, 1981, 21(2), 227-236.

[22] Thanos, S; Kacza, J; Seeger, J; Mey, J. Old dyes for new scopes: the phagocytosis-dependent long-term fluorescence labelling of microglial cells in vivo. *Trends Neurosci.*, 1994, 17(5), 177-182.

[23] Ng, TF; Streilein, JW. Light-induced migration of retinal microglia into the subretinal space. *Invest Ophthalmol Vis Sci.*, 2001, 42(13), 3301-3310.

[24] Dunaief, JL; Dentchev, T; Ying, GS; Milam, AH. The role of apoptosis in age-related macular degeneration. *Arch Ophthalmol.*, 2002, 120(11), 1435-1442.

[25] Bunt-Milam, AH; Saari, JC. Immunocytochemical localization of two retinoid-binding proteins in vertebrate retina. *J Cell Biol.*, 1983, 97(3), 703-712.

[26] Berson, EL; Rosner, B; Sandberg, MA *et al.* Vitamin A supplementation for retinitis pigmentosa. *Arch Ophthalmol.*, 1993, 111(11), 1456-1459.

[27] Hasson, T; Heintzelman, MB; Santos-Sacchi, J; Corey, DP; Mooseker, MS. Expression in cochlea and retina of myosin VIIa, the gene product defective in Usher syndrome type 1B. *Proc Natl Acad Sci.*, USA., 1995, 92(21), 9815-9819.

[28] Weil, D; Blanchard, S; Kaplan, J; et al. Defective myosin VIIA gene responsible for Usher syndrome type 1B. *Nature.*, 1995, 374(6517), 60-61.

[29] McLaughlin, ME; Sandberg, MA; Berson, EL; Dryja, TP. Recessive mutations in the gene encoding the beta-subunit of rod phosphodiesterase in patients with retinitis pigmentosa. *Nat Genet.*, 1993, 4(2), 130-134.

[30] Huang, SH; Pittler, SJ; Huang, X; Oliveira, L; Berson, EL; Dryja, TP. Autosomal recessive retinitis pigmentosa caused by mutations in the alpha subunit of rod cGMP phosphodiesterase. *Nat Genet.*, 1995, 11(4), 468-471.

[31] Zack, DJ. Ocular gene therapy. From fantasy to foreseeable reality. *Arch Ophthalmol.*, 1993, 111(11), 1477-1479.

[32] Bennett, J; Tanabe, T; Sun, D; et al. Photoreceptor cell rescue in retinal degeneration (rd) mice by in vivo gene therapy. *Nat Med.*, 1996, 2(6), 649-654.

[33] Bennett, J; Wilson, J; Sun, D; Forbes, B; Maguire, A. Adenovirus vector-mediated in vivo gene transfer into adult murine retina. *Invest Ophthalmol Vis Sci.*, 1994, 35(5), 2535-2542.

[34] Maguire, AM; Simonelli, F; Pierce, EA *et al.* Safety and efficacy of gene transfer for Leber's congenital amaurosis. *N Engl J Med.*, 2008, 358(21), 2240-2248.

[35] Naik, R; Mukhopadhyay, A; Ganguli, M. Gene delivery to the retina: focus on non-viral approaches. *Drug Discov Today.*, 2009, 14(5-6), 306-315.

[36] Park, TK; Wu, Z; Kjellstrom, S *et al.* Intravitreal delivery of AAV8 retinoschisin results in cell type-specific gene expression and retinal rescue in the Rs1-KO mouse. *Gene Ther.*, 2009.

[37] Cottet, S; Schorderet, DF. Mechanisms of apoptosis in retinitis pigmentosa. *Curr Mol Med.*, 2009, 9(3), 375-383.

[38] Takano, Y; Ohguro, H; Dezawa, M; et al. Study of drug effects of calcium channel blockers on retinal degeneration of rd mouse. *Biochem Biophys Res Commun.*, 2004, 313(4), 1015-1022.

[39] Perche, O; Doly, M; Ranchon-Cole, I. Transient protective effect of caspase inhibitors in RCS rat. *Exp Eye Res.*, 2008, 86(3), 519-527.

[40] Doonan, F; Donovan, M; Cotter, TG. Caspase-independent photoreceptor apoptosis in mouse models of retinal degeneration. *J Neurosci.*, 2003, 23(13), 5723-5731.

[41] Doonan, F; Donovan, M; Cotter, TG. Activation of multiple pathways during photoreceptor apoptosis in the rd mouse. *Invest Ophthalmol Vis Sci.*, 2005, 46(10), 3530-3538.

[42] Doonan, F; Cotter, TG. Apoptosis: a potential therapeutic target for retinal degenerations. *Curr Neurovasc Res.*, 2004, 1(1), 41-53.

[43] Donovan, M; Cotter, TG. Caspase-independent photoreceptor apoptosis in vivo and differential expression of apoptotic protease activating factor-1 and caspase-3 during retinal development. *Cell Death Differ.*, 2002, 9(11), 1220-1231.

[44] Miki, T; Kiyonaka, S; Uriu, Y *et al.* Mutation associated with an autosomal dominant cone-rod dystrophy CORD7 modifies RIM1-mediated modulation of voltage-dependent Ca2+ channels. *Channels (Austin).*, 2007, 1(3), 144-147.

[45] Faktorovich, EG; Steinberg, RH; Yasumura, D; Matthes, MT; LaVail, MM. Photoreceptor degeneration in inherited retinal dystrophy delayed by basic fibroblast growth factor. *Nature.*, 1990, 347(6288), 83-86.

[46] Perry, J; Du, J; Kjeldbye, H; Gouras, P. The effects of bFGF on RCS rat eyes. *Curr Eye Res.*, 1995, 14(7), 585-592.

[47] Joly, S; Lange, C; Thiersch, M; Samardzija, M; Grimm, C. Leukemia inhibitory factor extends the lifespan of injured photoreceptors in vivo. *J Neurosci.*, 2008, 28(51), 13765-13774.

[48] Yang, Y; Mohand-Said, S; Danan, A *et al.* Functional cone rescue by RdCVF protein in a dominant model of retinitis pigmentosa. *Mol Ther.*, 2009, 17(5), 787-795.

[49] Gregory-Evans, K; Chang, F; Hodges, MD; Gregory-Evans, CY. Ex vivo gene therapy using intravitreal injection of GDNF-secreting mouse embryonic stem cells in a rat model of retinal degeneration. *Mol Vis.*, 2009, 15, 962-973.

[50] MacDonald, IM; Sauve, Y; Sieving, PA. Preventing blindness in retinal disease: ciliary neurotrophic factor intraocular implants. *Can J Ophthalmol.*, 2007, 42(3), 399-402.

[51] Lin, N; Fan, W; Sheedlo, HJ; Turner, JE. Basic fibroblast growth factor treatment delays age-related photoreceptor degeneration in Fischer 344 rats. *Exp Eye Res.*, 1997, 64(2), 239-248.

[52] Emerich, DF; Thanos, CG. NT-501: an ophthalmic implant of polymer-encapsulated ciliary neurotrophic factor-producing cells. *Curr Opin Mol Ther.*, 2008, 10(5), 506-515.

[53] Gupta, N; Brown, KE; Milam, AH. Activated microglia in human retinitis pigmentosa, late-onset retinal degeneration, and age-related macular degeneration. *Exp Eye Res.*, *2003*, 76(4), 463-471.

[54] Ni, YQ; Xu, GZ; Hu, WZ; Shi, L; Qin, YW; Da, CD. Neuroprotective effects of naloxone against light-induced photoreceptor degeneration through inhibiting retinal microglial activation. *Invest Ophthalmol Vis Sci.*, 2008, 49(6), 2589-2598.

[55] Sasahara, M; Otani, A; Oishi, A; et al. Activation of bone marrow-derived microglia promotes photoreceptor survival in inherited retinal degeneration. *Am J Pathol.*, 2008, 172(6), 1693-1703.

[56] Humayun, MS; de Juan, E Jr.; del Cerro, M; et al. Human neural retinal transplantation. *Invest Ophthalmol Vis Sci.*, 2000, 41(10), 3100-3106.

[57] Radtke, ND; Aramant, RB; Petry, HM; Green, PT; Pidwell, DJ; Seiler, MJ. Vision improvement in retinal degeneration patients by implantation of retina together with retinal pigment epithelium. *Am J Ophthalmol.*, 2008, 146(2), 172-182.

Chapter V

Mutational Analysis of Rho and Rds Genes in Patients with Retinitis Pigmentosa from Volga-Ural Region of Russia

Lilya U. Dzhemileva[*], Elvira R. Grinberg, Ildar S. Zaidullin and Elza K. Khusnutdinova

[1] Institute of Biochemistry and Genetics Ufa Scientific Center Russian Academy of Science, Russia, Ufa, 450054, Prospect Octyabrya 71.

Abstract

We identified mutations in the RHO and RDS genes in patients with autosomal dominant and sporadic forms of retinitis pigmentosa (RP) from Volga-Ural region of Russia. The 5 exons of RHO and 3 exons of RDS genes were analyzed for sequence changes by single-strand conformation polymorphism (SSCP) and direct sequencing. Patients were examined clinically and with visual function tests. We detected known mutation Pro347Leu and novel mutation Arg252Pro and two polymorphisms IVS1+10g>a, IVS3+4c>t in RHO gene. There were statistically significant differences in allele and genotype frequencies of

[*] Corresponding author: +73472356088 (Tel), +73472356088 (Fax), E-mail Dzhemilev@anrb.ru

sequence change IVS3+4c>t of RHO gene in affected patients with RP and in controls. According to our data, this polymorphism is likely to be pathogenic. Recently were reported 16 possible combinations of the exon 3 RDS gene SNPs and detected four from 16 possible combinations (minihaplotypes): $G^{1147}A^{1166}G^{1250}C^{1291}$ (I), $C^{1147}A^{1166}A^{1250}C^{1291}$ (II), $C^{1147}G^{1166}A^{1250}C^{1291}$ (III) and $G^{1147}A^{1166}G^{1250}T^{1291}$ (IV). Telmer C.A. 2003 established that minihaplotype $C^{1147}A^{1166}A^{1250}C^{1291}$ (II) was linked to the mutation IVS2+3a>t. Sequencing results for variant positions in exon 3 RDS gene in RP patients from Volga-Ural region showed all four minihaplotypes described above and minihaplotype $C^{1147}A^{1166}A^{1250}T^{1291}$ (V). Our study determined that minihaplotype $C^{1147}A^{1166}A^{1250}C^{1291}$ (II) isn't linked to mutation IVS2+3a>t in adRP and sporadic RP patients from Volga-Ural region. To optimize the DNA diagnostics of retinitis pigmentosa, it is necessary to analyze patients from various ethnic groups. Our study helps in molecular characterization of RP in Russia.

Keywords: Retinitis pigmentosa, RHO gene, RDS gene, mutation analysis, polymerase chain reaction, single-strand conformation polymorphism analysis, direct DNA sequence analysis.

Introduction

Inherited retinal degenerative diseases are characterized by the progressive loss of photoreceptor cells through apoptosis [1]. Among them, retinitis pigmentosa, the most common hereditary cause of blindness, comprises a clinically and genetically heterogeneous group of retinal disorders [2]. It affects about one in 5 000 individuals worldwide [3]. Common clinical features include a progressive loss of night vision, leading to night blindness; peripheral-visual-field loss; abnormalities present on electroretinography; tunnel vision; optic-disk pallor; attenuation of the retinal blood vessels; intraretinal pigment deposition; and progressive visual handicap [4,5,6]. RP can be inherited in autosomal dominant, autosomal recessive, X-linked or digenic models. RP can present either alone or as a syndromic disorder [7]. Our study focused on patients with nonsyndromic forms of these diseases. RP is a paradigm of monogenic diseases with extremely high genetic heterogeneity: 11 genes and one locus were reported for autosomal dominant RP, 17 genes and five loci for autosomal recessive RP, and two genes and two loci for X-linked RP. The known genes can be classified into metabolic groups according to the encoded protein: visual transduction, visual cycle, transcription factors, structural proteins, spliceosome complex and cellular traffic, indicating the high level of specialization of photoreceptors and of the retinal pigment epithelium [8].

In the autosomal dominant form (adRP), which comprises about 25% of total cases, approximately 30% of families have mutations in the gene encoding the rod photoreceptor-specific protein rhodopsin. This is the transmembrane protein which, when photoexcited, initiates the visual transduction cascade. Rhodopsin is considered to be a prototypical G protein-coupled receptor. As a representative G protein-coupled receptor, rhodopsin is an integral membrane protein composed of three distinct regions: the intracellular (cytoplasmic), transmembrane, and extracellular (intradiscal) regions [9]. The RHO gene maps to human chromosome 3q21, consists of 5 exons. Up to 150 mutations, spanning the entire coding region, have so far been identified [10].

Another gene associated with adRP is the RDS gene coding for periferin/RDS. RDS gene encode a cell surface glycoprotein found in the outer segment of both rod and cone photoreceptor cells. It may function as an adhesion molecule involved in stabilization and compaction of outer segment disks or in the maintenance of the curvature of the rim. Its mutations account for 2-4% of cases of adRP [11]. 43 nucleotide sequence variants have been described in the human RDS gene. Out of this, 39 have been found to be associated with retinal phenotypes, including 16 associated with adRP [12].

Since RHO and RDS gene mutations have been shown to account for 1/3 of the adRP cases, these genes were chosen for screening of disease causing mutations. In this report, we describe mutation analysis of the RHO and RDS genes in patients with autosomal dominant and sporadic forms of retinitis pigmentosa from Volga-Ural region of Russia.

The Volga–Ural region of Russia, which is at the boundary between Europe and Asia, is of particular interest, because its ethnic populations mostly belong to the Turkic, Finno-Ugric, and Slavonic linguistic groups and have complex ethno genesis and specific features of the gene pool and genetic structure; and combine the Caucasian and Mongoloid components in various proportions. To optimize the DNA diagnostics of retinitis pigmentosa, it is necessary to analyze RHO and RDS genes for mutations in patients from various ethnic groups.

Molecular Aspects of in Patients with Retinitis Pigmentosa from the Volga–Ural Region

Among 123 unrelated RP patient's inheritance could be determined in 50.4% of the cases including dominant autosomic 30.1%, recessive autosomic 18.7%, and X-linked cases 1.6% while it could not be confirmed in 49.6% of the cases (sporadic cases).

37 cases showing adRP were chosen for mutation screening of RHO and RDS genes. Patients with dominant retinitis pigmentosa had at least one affected parent and all affected siblings. 61 patients with isolate RP also were included in this study; they had no affected relatives and were not the offspring of a consanguineous mating. All patients reside in the Volga-Ural region, Russia. Ophthalmic examinations of patients included slit lamp biomicroscopy, assessment of visual acuity, color perception, and visual fields; electroretino-grams (ERGs); and ascertainment of family history was performed in the Research Institute of Eye Diseases. All patients had progressive forms of retinitis pigmentosa based on history, clinical findings, and ERG abnormalities. 130 control individuals from the same ethnic background as the RP patients had no known blood relatives with a hereditary retinal degeneration and no symptoms of visual malfunction.

All patients gave informed consent to participate in the study, which adhered to the tenets of the Declaration of Helsinki and was approved by the Institutional Review Boards of the Institute of Biochemistry and Genetics and Research Institute of Eye Diseases.

DNA was prepared from whole blood using standard methods. Genomic DNA was isolated from 10 ml of peripheral blood by phenol–chloroform extraction [13], dissolved in water, and stored at −20°C. After polymerase chain reaction (PCR), the single-strand conformation polymorphism analysis (SSCP) [14] was used to screen for point mutations and other small-scale sequence changes within 5 exons of the RHO gene and 3 exons of the RDS gene. Exon 1 of RHO gene is a relatively large exon and was amplified in two overlapping segments; exons 2, 3, 4 and 5 were amplified in a single amplicon each. Exon 1 of RDS gene is large too and was amplified in three overlapping segments); exons 2 and 3 were amplified in a single amplicon each. Oligonucleotide primer pairs were chosen to amplify DNA of all 5 exons of the RHO gene, 3 exons of the RDS [15].

Amplification conditions were as follows. RHO gene sequences (all exons): 30 cycles of denaturing at 94°C for 1 min, annealing at 59°C for 1 min and extension at 72°C for 1 min. RDS sequences : 30 cycles of denaturing at 94°C for 1 min, annealing at 61°C for 1 min (exons 1.1, 1.2, 1.3, 2) or 55°C (exon 3) and extension at 72°C for 1 min. Direct DNA sequence analysis (ABI PRISM 310 (Applied Biosystems)) with the same primer pairs used for PCR amplification was used to confirm suspected DNA sequence changes. Sequence variations expected to affect protein sequence or expression were evaluated further by recruiting the relatives of the patients with adRP to participate in a study to determine whether the variant alleles cosegregated with the disease. For this purpose, leukocyte DNA samples from the relatives were analyzed by single strand conformation polymorphism or direct genomic sequencing for the presence of the variant sequences.

Table 1. Summary of RHO and RDS sequence variants detected in patients with RP from Volga-Ural region, Russia.

Gene	Exon / intron	Mutation / polymorphism	Nucleotide substitution	Amino acid substitution	Status	Patients allele frequency (adRP)	Patients allele frequency (sporadic RP)	Controls allele frequency
RHO	IVS1	IVS1+10g>a	G>A	-	Hetero	-	0.008	-
RHO	IVS3	IVS3+4c>t	C>T	-	Hetero	0.31	0.34	0.06
RHO	4	R252P	G>C	Arg252Pro	Hetero	0.01	-	-
RHO	5	P347L	C>T	Pro347Leu	Hetero	0.01	-	-
RDS	1	V106V	T>C	Val106Val	Hetero/Homo	0.3	0.2	0.34
RDS	3	E304Q	G>C	Glu304Gln	Hetero/Homo	0.28	0.27	0.54
RDS	3	K310R	G>A	Lys310Arg	Hetero/Homo	0.8	0.86	0.82
RDS	3	G338D	A>G	Gly338Asp	Hetero/Homo	0.66	0.73	0.85
RDS	3	1054 c>t	c>t	-	Hetero/Homo	0.8	0.8	0.43
RDS	3'UTR	1426g>a	g>a	-	Hetero	0.15	0.25	0.23

Table 2. Summary of RDS gene exon 3 patients and control individuals genotypes.

1147* (910)**	1166* (929)**	1250* (1013)**	1291* (1054)**	Minihaplotype Allele	Controls genotypes frequency (N=130)	Patients with adRP genotypes frequency (N=37)	χ^2, df=1	p	Patients with sporadic RP genotypes frequency (N=61)	χ^2, df=1	p
G/G	A/A	G/G	C/C	I, I	0.03 (N=4)	0	—	—	0	—	—
C/C	A/A	A/A	C/C	II, II	0	0.05 (n=2)	—	—	0	—	—
C/C	G/G	A/A	C/C	III, III	0.16 (N=21)	0.11 (n=4)	0.29	0.59	0.13 (n=8)	0.11	0.74
G/G	A/A	G/G	T/T	IV, IV	0.44 (N=57)	0.63 (n=23)	3.17	0.08	0.69 (n=42)	9.4	0.002
C/G	G/A	A/G	C/T	III, IV	0.37 (N=48)	0.11 (n=4)	7.98	0.005	0.02 (n=1)	25.3	0.0001
C/C	A/A	A/A	C/T	II, V	0	0.05 (n=2)	—	—	0.1 (n=6)	—	—
C/G	A/A	A/G	C/T	II, IV	0	0.05 (n=2)	—	—	0.06 (n=4)	—	—

* number of nucleotide positions is given according to GenBank

** number of nucleotide positions is given according to Retina International's Mutation Database.

To determine the relative contribution of RHO and RDS mutations to the causes of adRP and sporadic RP, we screened a group of 98 unrelated patients using SSCP analysis and further direct DNA sequencing. The results of our research are presented in Table 1.

The RHO gene mutation Pro347Leu changing the preterminal amino acid of the rhodopsin molecule has already been described [16, 17]. It is relatively frequent and tends to be associated with severe forms of RP. It's present in 2 adRP patients in 1 family and absence in unaffected individuals. This mutation was identified in 1 out of 37 adRP probands tested in heterozygous form, thus; its prevalence appears to be around 0.01. Patients with retinitis pigmentosa produced by rhodopsin mutations affecting the C terminus have more rapidly progressing disease with respect to visual field loss and ERG amplitude decline than patients with mutations affecting other regions. This suggests that impaired sorting and vectorial transport of rhodopsin (mutations affecting the C terminus) are associated with a more rapid rate of photoreceptor degeneration than defects associated with impaired folding (i.e., the globule mutations) or the abnormal formation of a functional pocket for the binding of vitamin A (i.e., the plug mutations) [18].

RHO gene mutation Arg252Pro was detected in 3 adRP patients in 1 family. It was absent in unaffected individuals. Mutation Arg252Pro has not been described before. Established that residue 252 is included in transducin's binding region (residues 231-252) [19]. Therefore, amino acid substitution in this region may influence on activation transducin in visual cascade. Another mutation Lys248Leu in the same region has been shown to prevent activation transducin in vitro [20]. So, mutation R252P of RHO gene is likely to be pathogenic. Therefore, further analysis of others RP-associated genes in that family is necessary in order to clarify the fenotyping manifestation of this mutation and its possible association with adRP.

Also we detected two sequence changes in RHO gene. One of them is known sequence change IVS3+4c>t (http://www. retina-international.org/sci-news/rhomut.htm; Retina International's Mutation Database). There were statistically significant differences in allele and genotype frequencies of sequence change IVS3+4c>t of RHO gene in affected patients with RP 0.31 and 0.34 (adRP and sporadic RP) and in controls 0.06 (χ^2_1=17.85, p<0.001; χ^2_2=21.34, p<0.001). So, according to our data, this polymorphism is likely to be pathogenic. It may be associated with disturbance or slow down of splicing process. Another sequence change IVS1+10g>a is in the intron region and It seems most probable not associated with RP.

As evident from table 1, we couldn't find any mutations in RDS gene. The most frequent nucleotide sequence changes in the RDS gene exon 3 identified in the adRP and sporadic RP patients from Volga-Ural region were Lys310Arg and Gly338Asp. Also, in exon 3 was detected sequences change in codon 304 Glu304Gln. Although each of them leads to an amino acid substitution, no correlation with the clinical manifestation of photoreceptor disorder has been found yet [21, 22]. Thus, they can be considered as neutral amino acid polymorphisms. Another sequence anomaly of RDS gene exon 1, silent changes within codon 106 (Val106Val) was interpreted as nonpathogenic polymorphism because it was predicted to have no effect on the encoded protein. Sequence changes 3'UTR 1054c>t and 3'UTR 1426g>a are in uncoding region of exon 3 of *RDS* gene, consequently they are nonpathogenic too [22].

Recently were reported 16 possible combinations of the exon 3 SNPs (Glu304Gln, Lys310Arg, Gly338Asp and 3'UTR 1054c>t) and detected four from 16 possible combinations (minihaplotypes): $G^{1147}A^{1166}G^{1250}C^{1291}$ (allele I), $C^{1147}A^{1166}A^{1250}C^{1291}$ (allele II), $C^{1147}G^{1166}A^{1250}C^{1291}$ (allele III) and $G^{1147}A^{1166}G^{1250}T^{1291}$ (allele IV), also were identified five genotypes consist of four alleles described before [23].

The minihaplotype $G^{1147}A^{1166}G^{1250}C^{1291}$ (allele I) corresponds to the published mRNA sequence (GenBank NM_000322) and the $C^{1147}G^{1166}A^{1250}C^{1291}$ minihaplotype (allele III) corresponds to the RDS/peripherin genomic sequence (GenBank AL049843). Sequencing results for variant positions in exon 3 RDS gene in RP patients from Volga-Ural region showed all four minihaplotypes described above and minihaplotype $C^{1147}A^{1166}A^{1250}T^{1291}$ (allele V). Table 2 shows the *RDS* gene exon 3 genotypes of adRP, sporadic RP and control individuals from Volga-Ural region analyzed.

As evident from table 2 the most frequent genotype in the RDS gene exon 3 identified in the adRP and sporadic RP patients from Volga-Ural region was $G/G^{1147}A/A^{1166}G/G^{1250}T/T^{1291}$ (allele IV in homozygous form), also it was the most frequent genotype in the RDS/PRPH2 gene exon 3 in control individuals too. Three genotypes $C/C^{1147}A/A^{1166}A/A^{1250}C/C^{1291}$ (allele II in homozygous form), $C/C^{1147}A/A^{1166}A/A^{1250}C/T^{1291}$ (alleles II, V), $C/G^{1147}A/A^{1166}A/G^{1250}C/T^{1291}$ (alleles II, IV) were not found in control individuals and contained minihaplotype $C^{1147}A^{1166}A^{1250}C^{1291}$ (allele II). Telmer C.A. in 2003 reported that minihaplotype $C^{1147}A^{1166}A^{1250}C^{1291}$ (allele II) was linked to the mutation IVS2+3a>t in 12 unrelated patients with macular degeneration phenotypes.

This substitution (IVS2+3a>t) is in the 5' splice site of intron 2 of RDS gene and was reported previously in an independent pedigree [24]. Sequence analysis of exon 2 of RDS gene in all adRP and sporadic RP patients from Volga-Ural region with genotypes contained minihaplotype $C^{1147}A^{1166}A^{1250}C^{1291}$ (allele II) didn't show any sequences changes in the 5' splice site of intron 2 RDS gene. So, according to our data, minihaplotype $C^{1147}A^{1166}A^{1250}C^{1291}$ (allele II) isn't linked to mutation IVS2+3a>t in adRP and sporadic RP patients from Volga-Ural region.

The true prevalence of rhodopsin and peripherin mutations and polymorphisms among patients with RP from Volga-Ural region may be a bit higher than described above because the screening method (SSCP) may miss approximately 10% of point mutations [25, 26, 27]. On the other hand all currently known genes do not represent more than 50% of RP cases, suggesting that many genes remain to be discovered [8]. So the cause of retinitis pigmentosa in patients from Volga-Ural region may be mutations in another genes associated with RP even have not been discovered yet. Identification of genes may help in diagnosis and in genetic counseling RP in particular in Volga-Ural region, especially in simplex cases with retinitis pigmentosa. Also in latter condition, molecular diagnosis will be necessary to rationalize future treatments.

Acknowledgements

This work was supported by the Russian Foundations for Human Research (projects nos. 08-06-84602a/U, MD-3049.2007.7, and MK-2575.2008.4).

References

[1]   Fain, GL. Why photoreceptors die (and why they don't). *BioEssays*, 2006, 28(4), 344-354.

[2]   Rivolta, C; Sharon, D; DeAngelis, MM; Dryja, TP. Retinitis pigmentosa and allied diseases: numerous diseases, genes, and inheritance patterns. *Hum Mol Genet.*, 2002, 11(10), 1219-1227.

[3]   Weleber, RG; Gregory-Evans, K. *Retinitis pigmentosa and allied disorders.*, In S. J. Ryan (Ed.), Retina. Mosby, St. Louis, 362-470, 2001.

[4]   Dryja, T; Li, T. Molecular genetics of retinitis pigmentosa. *Hum Mol Genet.*, 1995, 4, 1739-1743.

[5]   Herse, P. Retinitis pigmentosa: visual function and multidisciplinary management. *Clin Exp Optom.*, 2005, 88(5), 335-350.

[6]   Hamel, C. Retinitis pigmentosa. *Orphanet Journal of Rare Diseases.*, 2006, 22, 1-40.

[7]   Hims, MM; Diager, SP; Inglehearn, CF. Retinitis pigmentosa: genes proteins and prospects. *Dev Ophthalmol.*, 2003, 37, 109-125.

[8]   Maubaret, S; Hamel, CP. Genetics of retinitis pigmentosa: metabolic classification and phenotype/genotype correlations. *Jr Fr Ophthalmol.*, 2005, 28(1), 1-92.

[9]   Sakmar, TP. Rhodopsin: a prototypical G protein-coupled receptor. *Prog Nucleic Acids Res Mol Biol.*, 1998, 59, 1-3.

[10]   Garriga, P; Manosa, J. The eye photoreceptor protein rhodopsin. Structural implications for retinal disease. *FEBS Letters.*, 2002, 528, 17-22.

[11]   Sung, CH; Davenport, CM; Hennessey, JC. Rhodopsin mutations in autosomal dominant retinitis pigmentosa. *Proc Natl Acad Sci.*, USA., 1991, 88, 6481-6584.

[12]   Keen, TJ; Inglehearn, CF. Mutations and polymorphisms in the human peripherin-RDS gene and their involvement in inherited retinal degeneration. *Hum Mutat.*, 1996, 8, 297-303.

[13]   Mathew, CC. Methods in Molecular Biology. *Humana press.*, 1984 4, 31-34.

[14]   Orita, M; Iwahana, H; Kanazawa, H; Sekya, T. Detection of polymorphism of human DNA by gel electrophoresis as single cell conformation polymorphism. *Proc Natl Acad Sci.*, 1989 86, 2766-2770.

[15]   Van Lith-Verhoeven, JC; Cremers, FP; Van den Helm, B. Genetic heterogeneity of butterfly-shaped pigment dystrophy of the fovea. *Mol Vis.*, 2003, 9, 138-143.

[16]   Dryja, T; McGee, T; Hahn, L. Mutations within the rhodopsin gene in patients with autosomal dominant retinitis pigmentosa. *New Eng J Med.*, 1990, 323, 1302-1307.

[17]   Zhang, XL; Liu, M; Meng, XH; et al. Mutational analysis of the rhodopsin gene in Chinese ADRP families by conformation sensitive gel electrophoresis. *Life Sci.*, 2006, 78(13), 1494-1498.

[18] Berson, E; Rosner, B; Weigel-DiFranco, C; Dryja, T. & Sandberg, M. Disease progression in patients with dominant retinitis pigmentosa and rhodopsin mutations. *Invest Ophthalmol Vis Sci.*, 2002, 43(9), 3027-3036.

[19] Franke, RR; Sakmar, TP; Graham, RM; Khorana, HG. Structure and Function in Rhodopsin. Studies of the interaction between the rhodopsin cytoplasmic domain and trunsdusin. *J Biol Chem.*, 1992, 267(21), 14767-14774

[20] Franke, RR; Sakmar, TP; Oprian, DD; Khorana, HG. A single amino acid substitution in rhodopsin (Lys248Leu) prevents activation of transducin. *J Biol Chem.*, 1988, 263, 2119-2122.

[21] Jordan, SA; Farrar, GJ; Kenna, P; Humphries, P. Polymorphic variation within 'conserved' sequences at the 3' end of the human RDS gene with results in amino acid substitutions. *Hum Mutat.*, 1992, 1, 240-247.

[22] Kucinskas, V; Payne, AM; Ambrasiene, D; Jurgelevicius, V; Steponaviciute, D; Arciulienen, JV; Daktaraviciene, E; Bhattacharya, S. Molecular genetic study of autosomal dominant retinitis pigmentosa in Lithuanian patients. *Hum Hered.*, 1999, 49, 71-74.

[23] Telmer, CA; Retchless, AR; Kinsey, AD. Detection and Assignment of Mutations and Minihaplotypes in Human DNA Using Peptide Mass Signature Genotyping (PMSG): Application to the Human RDS/Peripherin Gene. *Genom Res.*, 2003, 13, 1944-1951.

[24] Sullivan, LS; Daiger, SP. Inherited retinal degeneration: exceptional genetic and clinical heterogeneity. *Mol Med Today.*, 1996, 2, 380-388.

[25] Condie, A; Eeles, R; Borresen, A; Coles, C; Cooper, C. & Prosser, J. Detection of point mutations in the p53 gene: comparison of single-strand conformation polymorphism, constant denaturant gel electrophoresis, and hydroxylamine and osmium tetroxide techniques. *Hum Mutat.*, 1993, 2, 58-66.

[26] Hayashi, K; Yandell, DW. How sensitive is PCR-SSCP? *Hum Mutat.*, 1993, 2, 338-346.

[27] Sheffield, VC; Beck, JS; Kwitek, AE; Sandstrom, DW; Stone, EM. The sensitivity of single-strand conformation polymorphism analysis for the detection of single base substitutions. *Genomics.*, 1993, 16, 325-332.

[28] Dryja, T; Hahn, L; Cowley, G; McGee, T. & Berson, E. Mutation spectrum of the rhodopsin gene among patients with autosomal dominant retinitis pigmentosa. *Proc Natl Acad Sci.*, USA., 1991, 88, 9370-9374.

In: Reginitis Pigmentosa: Causes, Diagnosis…   ISBN: 978-1-60876-884-4
Editors: M. Baert, et al. pp. 139-190   © 2010 Nova Science Publishers, Inc.

Chapter VI

Physiopathology of Retinal Degeneration in Rd1 Mouse Model of Retinitis Pigmentosa: TGF-B1, Proteinases and Oxidative Stress Mechanisms[*]

Satpal Ahuja[† a], *Poonam Ahuja-Jensen*[b],
A. Romeo Caffe´[a, c], *Magnus Abrahamson*[d],
Per Ekstroma and Theo van Veen[a, e]

[a] Ophthalmology Division, Department of Clinical Sciences, BMC B-13,
Klinikgatan 26, Lund University, SE-22184 Lund, Sweden.
[b] Vårdcentralen (Kommune Health Center), Kvarngatan 21,
SE-24431 Kävlinge, Sweden.
[c] Bombaydreef 61, Utrecht, The Netherlands.
[d] Department of Laboratory Medicine.

[*] A version of this chapter was also published in Retinal Degeneration: Causes, Diagnosis and Treatment, edited by Robert B. Catlin, Nova Science Publishers. It was submitted for appropriate modifications in an effort to encourage wider dissemination of research.
[†] Corresponding author: Satpal Ahuja, Ophthalmology Division , Department of Clinical Sciences, BMC B-13, Klinikgatan 26, Lund University, SE-22184 Lund, Sweden, Email: sat_pal.ahuja@med.lu.se; Phone: +46 46 2220768, Fax: +46 46 2220774.

[e] University Eye Hospital, Schleistrasse 12-16,
D-72076 Tubingen, Germany.

Abstract

The rd1 (retinal degeneration) mouse retina shows degeneration homologous to a form of retinitis pigmentosa with a rapid loss of rod photoreceptors and deficiency of retinal blood vessels. Due to Pde6brd1 gene mutation, β subunit of phosphodiesterase (PDE) of rd1 retina has an inactive PDE which elevates cGMP and Ca2+ ions level. In vitro retinal explants provide a system close to the in vivo situation, so both approaches were used to compare the status of oxidative stress, transforming growth factor-β1

(TGF-β1), sialylation, galactosylation of proteoglycans, and different proteinases-endogenous inhibitors systems participating in extracellular matrix (ECM) remodeling/degeneration and programmed cell death (PCD)/apoptosis in wt and rd1 mouse retinas.

Proteins and desialylated sulfated glucosaminoglycan parts of proteoglycans in ECM of rd1 retina were, respectively, decreased and increased due to enhanced activities of proteinases. Desialylation increases the susceptibility of cells to phoagocytosis/ apoptosis, decreased neurogenesis and faulty guidance cues for synaptogenesis. In vivo activities of total proteinases, matrix metalloproteinase-9 (MMP-9) and cathepsin B were increased in rd1 retina on postnatal day 14 (PN14), -21 and -28, due to relatively lower levels of tissue inhibitor of MMPs (TIMP-1) and cystatin C, respectively. This corresponded with increased in vitro secretion of these proteinases by rd1 retina. Cells including end-feet of Mueller cells in degenerating rd1 retina showed intense immunolabeling for MMP-9, MMP-2/TIMP-1, TIMP-2 and cathepsin B/cystatin C, and proteinases pool was increased by Mueller cells. Intense immunolabeling of ganglion cell (RGC) layer for cathepsin B and of inner-plexiform layer of both PN2/PN7 rd1 and wt retinas indicated importance of cathepsin B in synaptogenesis and PCD of RGC.

Increased levels of TGF-β1 in vitro transiently increased the secretion of MMPs and cathepsins activities by wt explants which activate TGF-β1 and remodel the ECM for angiogenesis and ontogenetic PCD. Whereas, lower level of TGF-β1 and persistently higher activities of MMPs and cathepsins in rd1 retinas and conditioned medium, suggested that proteinases degraded TGF-β1 and ECM and caused retinal degeneration.

Lower activities of glutathione-S-transferase and glutathione-peroxidase in rd1 retina contribute to oxidative stress which damages membranes and increased the expression, release/secretion of proteinases relative to their endogenous inhibitors. Participation of oxidative stress in rd1 retinal degeneration was further confirmed from the partial protection of rd1 photoreceptors by in vitro and/or in vivo supplementation with glutathione-S-transferase or a combination of antioxidants namely lutein, zeaxanthin, α-lipoic acid and reduced-L-glutathione. Treatment with combination(s) of broad spectrum proteinase inhibitor(s) and antioxidants needs investigation.

Keywords: rd1 mouse retina/retinal explants, in vivo/in vitro TGF-β1, MMPs/TIMPs, cathepsins/cystatin C, proteoglycan levels, sialylation of proteoglycans.

Introduction

The Rd1 (Retinal Degeneration) Mouse Model of Retinitis Pigmentosa

Inherited retinal degenerations (IRD) affect around 1 in 3000 to 1 in 4000 of the population in the western countries. Retinitis pigmentosa is one of the IRD and refers to a group of inherited diseases due to autosomal dominant / recessive, X-linked mutations in least 30 genes (www.sph.uth.tmc.edu/retnet) and result in the death of rod photoreceptors followed by that of cones. Retina shows a common phenotype consisting of pigmented spots along with narrowing of retinal blood vessels [58]. During early stages, retinitis pigmentosa patients show night blindness after which there is a loss of peripheral vision, with a variable progression lasting for many years [96]. Due to a mutated $Pde6b^{rd1}$ gene for the β subunit of phosphodiesterase (PDE) the $rd1$ (retinal degeneration) mouse retina has an inactive PDE which elevates intracellular cGMP and Ca^{2+} ions levels [25, 39]. For instance, cGMP has been suggested to modify the expression of more than 60 genes involved in angiogenesis, turnover of extracellular matrix components (ECM), neural cell transcription, proliferation, apoptosis [88] and suppression of tissue inhibitor of matrix metalloproteinase-1 (TIMP-1) [93] and thus it indirectly increases the activity of matrix metalloproteinase (MMPs). The rod photoreceptor death in $rd1$ retina begins at postnatal day 9 (PN9), peaks at PN12 and by PN17 rods are in principle eliminated and the retina is left with only one row of cones [21]. As PDE mutation is also present in human patients, the *rd1* mouse is a relevant model for studies involving pathogenesis and treatment of retinitis pigmentosa [75]. The *rd1* mouse retina shows degenerative changes homologous to those observed in a form of retinitis pigmentosa but depicts rapid loss of rod photoreceptors and has retinal blood vessels deficiency [39, 74 and 110]. Deficiency of retinal blood vessels may decrease the number of endothelial cells and consequently lower the levels of neuroprotective brain-derived neurotrophic factor (BDNF) secreted by the endothelium [47] whose action requires polysialic acid sensitization of neurons in hippocampus [78]. Moreover, BDNF is degraded by proteinases [31, 38]. Thus *rd1* mouse and human patient retinas may also be deficient in BDNF and this view is supported by rescue of *rd1* photoreceptotor rods by BDNF plus ciliary neurotrophic factor (CNTF) [12].

Cellular Sources and Status of Transforming Growth Factor-B$_1$ (TGF-B$_1$), Proteinases, Proteinase Inhibitors and Oxidative Stress In Retinal Degeneration

Cellular sources

Cellular sources of different proteinases and their endogenous inhibitors during development of most of the diseases leading to retinal degeneration have not been identified [100]. Retinal cells form a network and are generally described as being organized into different layers. The component cells and cell processes constitute the following layers in which the proteinases and proteinase inhibitors can be visualized by immunoreactions. The outer- (OPL) and inner- (IPL) plexiform layers comprise of junctions between axon of photoreceptors with processes of integrating neurons namely bipolar and horizontal cells; and axons of bipolar cells and amacrine cells with processes of ganglion cells, respectively. The optic fiber layer comprises of axons of ganglion cells. The outer limiting membrane (OLM) represents occluding junctions separating outer nuclear layer (ONL) from the outer segments (OS) of photoreceptors. The OLM junctions are between plasma membranes (PM) of photoreceptor segments and the Mueller cells. Inner limiting membrane (ILM) represents fusion between the end feet processes of Mueller cells. The ONL, ganglion cell layer (GCL), and inner nuclear layer (INL) respectively comprise of cell bodies of photoreceptors, retinal ganglion cells (RGC) and integrating neurons, including horizontal, bipolar and amacrine cells. The combined proteinase activities of retinal resident and inflammatory cells as well as the vasculature are the likely sources of different proteinases and free radicals (Eye and retina; http://thalamus, and The retinal tunic; http://education.vetmed.vt.edu/curriculum/VM8054/EYE/ RETINA.HTM).

Proteinases and their endogenous inhibitors

Most of the studies on proteinases in retinal degeneration are represented by individual type of proteinases and little work has been carried out to determine the imbalance between proteinases and their endogenous inhibitors, or the interaction between different proteinases and their inhibitors to clarify their role in pathogenesis of retinal degenerations. In different tissues, six groups of proteinases such as aspartate (pepsin family), cysteine- (papain, caspase and calpain families), serine- (chymotrypsinogen family) glutamate- and threonine- proteinases and MMPs, have been described [30]. The MMPs, serine proteinases namely urokinase- (uPA) and tissue- (tPA) plasminogen activators and cysteine cathepsins and calpain are endogenously inhibited by TIMPs, plasminogen activator inhibitor-1 (PAI-1) / serpins, cystatin C and calpastatin respectively. In addition to these proteinases, proteasome degrade aberrant and other proteins, activate enzymes (Figure 1), promote damage to the RGC, modulate transport processes, cell signaling, immune response, wound healing and development [70, 73]. It has been reported that proteolytic activities up regulated during healing process to counteract the fibrosing process and there is interplay between matrix degrading proteinases, growth factors and adhesion molecules [122]. It is known that an imbalance in proteinases, proteasome and oxidative stress systems plays an important role in the pathogenesis of inflammatory and neurodegenerative diseases including retinal degenerations [6, 9, 34, 115 and J. Pietzsch, Signaling scissors: new perspectives on proteases, Horizon Symposia, 2003, www.nature.com/horizon/home.html]. MMP-9 is associated with degenerative diseases and its zymogen form namely pro-MMP-9 is activated by cathepsin G and inactivated by α-antichymotrypsin in skin. Thus activation of pro-MMP-9 and inactivation of α-antichymotrypsin are tightly associated in the degenerative process [123]. However, the proteinases involved in the inactivation of α-antichymotrypsin have not been identified. In addition to inhibiting MMPs, the proteinase inhibitors TIMPs have growth promoting effects [13, E. Smyth, The trouble with inhibitors, Horizon Symposia, 2003, www.nature.com/horizon/home.html], whereas cystatin C inhibitor of cathepsins increases the number of neural stem cells, modifies glial cell development, modulates neurodegenration and neurogenesis and prevents oxidative stress-induced death of PC12 cells [49, 81 and 91]. As a further complication in understanding these processes cystatin C and TIMPs have been shown to be degraded by serine proteinases and cysteine cathepsins, respectively in different tissues [1, 116] and result in the enhancement of cathepsin and MMPs activities. Cathepsin B and MMP-2 expression is upregulated by another MMP- an elastase [44]. Thus different proteinases and endogenous inhibitors show a hierarchy in their actions in different tissues which needs to be delineated for retinal degenerations, to understand their pathogenesis.

Microglia component of the glial cell population in the central nervous system (CNS) including retina are activated after injury to the neurons and perform their functions through nonspecific and specific limited proteolysis by intra- and extracellular proteinases [80]. Microglia are known to produce extracellular matrix (ECM), proteinases, cytokines including transforming growth factor-β (TGF-β), complement system components, reactive oxygen species (ROS) and nitric oxide (NO) [117]. By partial hydrolysis, proteinases generate as well as activate or inactivate bioactive molecules, irreversibly degrade ECM components and proteins of cells destined for elimination and lead to neuronal death [28, 80 and 117].

The activities of proteinases are regulated at different levels namely at gene level by regulation of transcription, at protein level by biosynthesis as inactive **zymogens' form, activation** by autoproteolysis or by other proteinases, metal ions, proteolysis of their inhibitors and inactivation by the inhibitors [24, 100, 104 and 105].

Sialylation of proteoglycans, TGF-β, proteinases and their inhibitors

In general the cellular sources and biochemical basis of the functions of TGF-β, **proteinases and** proteinase inhibitors in normal and degenerating retina are not well defined. Cytoplasm of retinal pigment epithelium (RPE), photoreceptors, Mueller cells, RGC, hyalocytes and cells associated with choroidal and retinal blood vessels of mammalian retina show one or more of the three isoforms of TGF-β, **which belongs** to the cytokine family [11]. These isoforms of TGF-β **are differentially involved in** the regulation of a variety of biological pathways, for instance TGF-β_1 inhibits glial cell proliferation including that promoted by basic fibroblast growth factor (bFGF) and protects neurons from ischemia, while TGF-β_1 and TGF–β_2 promote ingestion of rod outer segments by RPE [14]. TGF-β also mediates programmed cell death (PCD) in developing murine retina and regulates diverse cell functions like differentiation, proliferation, survival and migration including initiation of chemotaxis and angiogenesis for tissue repair [42]. In the ECM, TGF-β_1 driven cell differentiation is regulated by hyaluronan polysaccharides, which are oxidized by ROS and degraded during oxidative stress [76]. Such fragmentation of hyaluronan is inhibited by extracellular superoxide dismutase (SOD) which has a limited antioxidant action in the ECM [14].

ECM associated proteins and proteoglycans are further degraded by proteinases namely MMPs, cysteine cathepsins and serine proteinases [33, 92] leading to the accumulation of low molecular weight sulfated glycosaminoglycans (sGAG) in the ECM [6]. Activities of MMPs and serine proteinases such as tPA, uPA and plasmin are regulated by TIMPs and PAI-1 / serpins respectively and joint action of these proteinases and their physiological inhibitors determines the extent of angiogenesis and remodeling of ECM in tumors [73]. sGAG inhibits retinal migration of Mueller cells [98] which balance the pro- and antiangiogenic mediators in retina [114]. Furthermore, the extent of terminal sialylation or galactosylation of sGAG of proteoglycans determines whether a cell is prone to apoptosis and phagocytosis and the release of faulty guidance cues for axonal synaptogenesis between different types of neurons [43, 62, 67, 108 and 118]. Malfunctioning of mitochondria adversely affects the axonal transport and leads to defective synaptogenesis [35]. In addition to this, the binding of sialoprotein to MMP-2 alters inhibition kinetics of TIMPs [52] and consequently the MMPs proteinase activity.

TGF-β also plays a critical role in inducting the biosynthesis of ECM components such as collagens, fibronectin and proteoglycans [50, 69]. TGF-β is secreted as an inactive complex made up of TGF-β itself, a latency associated protein and TGF-β binding protein which links it to ECM through integrin $\alpha_3\beta_1$. The latter potentiates induction of MMP-9 for ECM remodeling in immortalized keratinocytes [60]. Latent TGF-β is released from ECM by proteinases associated with the cell surface and is activated by integrins to interact with TGF-β receptor-I and -II present in developing rat retina [69, 113]. Interaction between TGF-β and its receptor-I and –II has been observed, respectively from birth and embryonic day 17 through adulthood [113]. There are conflicting reports regarding the effects of TGF-β_1 on the type of tissue and MMP, their levels, secretion and activation [15, 92, 94, 99 and 111].

During development of lungs and emphysema in mice TGF-β_1 lowers MMP-12 and increases TIMP-1 [94, 111]. It is possible that under these conditions the lower activity of MMP-12 was due to inhibition by TIMP-1. TGF-β, tumor necrosis factor-α (TNF-α) and interleukine-1β (IL-1β) modulate the expression of cathepsins, MMP-1, MMP-3, and MMP-9 in several cell types and TGF-β_1 positively modulates the expression of MMP-2 and TIMP-1 in cultured human RPE cells [5, 30]. TGF-β_1 upregulates the expression of cystatin C. The latter antagonizes TGF-β_1 signaling in normal and cancer cells as well as regulates tissue inflammation [101]. Thus the balances between the activities of TGF-β and proteinase / proteinase inhibitor systems regulate each others' actions [31].

Oxidative stress

During mitochondrial utilization of molecular oxygen for production of ATP and reducing potential there is a concomitant generation of ROS and reactive nitrogen species (RNS) - the free radicals. Mitochondria are the major source of free radicals and elevation of the latter represents oxidative stress [71] which has been defined as a disruption of the balance in redox control and signaling pathways. This is evident from the reports and reviews on intra- and extracellular role of free radicals in biology and the CNS including retina [18, 37, 48, 54, 55 and 112]. ROS and RNS include free radicals of higher to intermediate reactivity. The free radicals - exemplified by superoxide (O_2^{*-}), hydrogen peroxide (H_2O_2), hydroxyl radical (OH^{*}), hydroxyl ion (OH^{-}) and NO - have short half life and high reactivity towards the molecules in their vicinity. H_2O_2 can permeate longer cytoplasmic distances than O_2^{*-} and has the potential to create a very reactive OH^{*} with disruptive changes in cellular locations like nucleus and the membranes [20]. When primary defense response involving antioxidants is inadequate, the free radicals modify the structure and function of biomolecules by oxidation of purine, pyrimidine bases in nucleic acids, unsaturated fatty acids components of membrane lipids and sulfahydryl (-SH) groups of cytosol and membrane associated proteins and disorganize DNA, RNA, proteins, lipids and membranes. In addition, the ROS and RNS themselves participate in the intracellular signaling processes [106] and may thus play important roles in health and disease.

Under physiological conditions ROS and RNS are removed by a number of scavenging systems (Figure 2) while under pathological conditions imbalance between the generation of free radicals and their removal favors their accumulation and consequently the oxidative stress. Due to profuse localized blood supply and exposure to light, the retina is predisposed to the generation of comparatively higher proportion of free radicals than other tissues and also possesses efficient scavenging systems. The accumulation of free radicals leading to oxidative stress is implicated in retinal degenerative diseases due to age related macular degeneration, diabetic retinopathy, retinitis pigmentosa, other inherited diseases and inflammation [96]. Moreover, blood vessel narrowing [58] and deficiency in the retina during retinitis pigmentosa [25, 39] creates hypoxia and consequently oxidative stress. Although antioxidants do not serve as a cure for neurodegeneration yet these have been shown to provide partial protection against harmful effects of free radicals [36, 57, 58 and 96].

Such protective effects in retina would prolong the period of better quality life of patients as the disease has a long duration for its progression to complete loss of vision.

Activated microglial cells and Mueller cells produce neuroactive substances like cytokines, proteinases and free radicals. The latter are products of NADPH oxidase (NOx) and induced nitric oxide synthetase (iNOS) which contribute to neuronal death during neurodegeneration. As a protective mechanism microglia cells extensively produce antioxidants like reduced glutathione (GSH) and the antioxidant enzymes (Figure 2) namely SOD, catalase, glutathione-peroxidase (GPx), glutathione-reductase (GR), glutathione-S-transferase (GST) and NADPH regenerating enzymes (NRE) [37]. GPx utilizes GSH, an intra- and extracellular antioxidant to detoxify peroxides [112].

Oxidative stress in retinitis pigmentosa contributes to rod and cone photoreceptor cell death without any regard for the type of mutation in the photoreceptors and leads to their loss [57]. Systemic injections of a mixture of antioxidants which included metalloporphyrin (MnTBAP, an SOD mimetic which protects against ROS), α-lipoic acid, ascorbic acid and α-tocopherol increased rhodopsin mRNA and promoted the survival of cones in *rd1* mice, while over expression of SOD-1 in mice, protected the retinas against oxidative stress [36, 57]. However, higher activity of SOD may also increase generation of H_2O_2, a free radical capable of generating more reactive free radicals OH* and OH⁻. In addition to SOD oxidases, NOS and NOx also contribute to oxidative stress [112]. Similarly from the *in vitro* and *in vivo* studies with *rd1* mice it was observed that GPx and GST deficiency at PN2 stage participate in retinal degeneration due to oxidative stress which was partially prevented *in vitro* by supplementation with GST [8]. Naturally occurring carotenoids namely zeaxanthin and lutein associated with photoreceptors in human retina are biologically active and protective against oxidative stress [102, 103]. Furthermore α-lipoic acid scavenges OH^* and singlet oxygen [82] and GSH, which is present in all tissues including different type of retinal cells, maintains normal redox status [41]. Structurally lipid soluble and water soluble antioxidants are different and have different biological activities suggesting that bolstering the endogenous defenses by a variety of antioxidants or antioxidant enzymes against oxidative stress forms a good strategy to slow down the process of retinal degeneration [96].

On the whole this chapter describes and reviews the sparsely investigated aspects of retinal physiopathology especially the information regarding the contribution of different cell types and the relative roles of TGF-β_1, sialylation of proteoglycans, different proteinases and their inhibitors in the physiopathological angiogenesis and photoreceptor cell death [6, 9, 86 and 100]. The revised interpretations presented herein were not possible for inclusion in the original individual reports [6, 7, 8, 9 and 96]. So the synthesis of our published and unpublished work [TGF-β_1 and secreted proteinases and their natural inhibitors] on retinal cell sources of proteinases and inhibitors, the biochemical basis of pathogenesis namely the role of TGF-β_1, extent of sialylation of sGAG, inter- and intra-proteinase type interactions and balance between different types of proteinases and their endogenous inhibitors; and rescue of photoreceptors by antioxidants and antioxidant enzymes in *rd1* mouse retinal degeneration have, therefore, been described.

Material and Methods

Animals and Tissues

Congenic wild type control mice of CH3 strain and homozygous retinal degeneration 1 (rd1/rd1) mice from the animal colonies at Lund University were used during these studies and were designated as *wt* and *rd1*, respectively. Day of birth was referred as postnatal day 0 (PN0). Pups below the age of PN7 were killed by decapitation, whereas older ones were asphyxiated on dry ice and then decapitated. All animals were treated in accordance with the European Communities Council Directive (86/609/EEC) and with the approval of Swedish National Animal Care and Ethics

Committee. The retinal explants were cultured *in vitro* because explants in such culture system show histological characteristics similar to those of age matched *wt* and *rd1* retinas developing *in vivo* [21].

Proteins, Sgag and Sialylation and Galactosylation of Sgag [See Reference 6 For Procedures]

Retinal extracts of PN2, -7, -14, -21 and -28 rd1 and wt retinas were prepared and analyzed for protein (Plus One 2-D Quant Kit, Amersham Pharmacia Biotech Sweden) and sGAG (with a kit from Wieslab AB, Lund, Sweden) contents. sGAG and proteoglycans in retinal extracts at different stages of development were fractionated by SDS-PAGE and then characterized by wheat germ agglutinin and peanut agglutinin lectins labeling for the extent of sialylation and galactosylation, respectively [6].

Cellular Sources and Levels Of TGF-B$_1$, Proteinases and their Endogenous Inhibitors in Retinal Extracts and Retinal Conditioned Medium (RCM)

Cellular sources [see references 6, 7 and 96 for procedures]
For spatial localization of MMP-2, MMP-9, cysteine cathepsin B, TIMP-1 and TIMP-2 commercial monoclonal primary antibodies were used and visualized by subsequent immunoreaction with an appropriate fluorescent / Texas Red labeled secondary antibody. However, cystatin C was localized with rabbit polyclonal antibodies raised by the Division of Clinical Chemistry and Pharmacology, Lund University and visualized as described for MMPs, cathepsin B and TIMPs. The PN9, -11 and -13 *wt* and *rd1* retinas were evaluated by immunohistochemistry for oxidatively damaged DNA.

Levels of proteinases and their inhibitors in retinal extracts and RCM [see references 6, 7 for procedures]
Retinas from PN2, -7, -14, -21 and -28 *wt* and *rd1* mice were dissected. Total proteinase activity in retinal extracts and retinal conditioned medium (RCM) from PN2 or PN7 explants was measured by fluorometry (Perkin Elmer, LS 50B Luminescence Spectrometer at 485 nm excitation and 530 nm

levels were quantified using immunocapture ELISA kits (Amersham Pharmacia Biotech, Uppsala, Sweden) and their endogenous inhibitors TIMP-1 and TIMP-2 were measured by sandwich ELISA kits (RandD Systems, Minneapolis, Minn., USA, for TIMPs) and as described in protocols provided by the manufacturers [6]. Cysteine cathepsins B and cathepsin L activity in the retinal extracts and RCM samples were measured by fluorometry using fluorogenic substrates namely carbobenzyloxy-L-phenyl-L-arginylamido-4-methyl coumarin and carbobenzyloxy-L-argnyl-L-arginylamido-4-methyl coumarin. N-methyl coumarin (NMec) was used as a standard [7]. Cathepsin S was measured after irreversible inactivation of other cathepsins at neutral pH. Cystatin C, an endogenous inhibitor of cathepsins was measured by ELISA [7].

RCM samples were also fractionated for protein profile by SDS-PAGE [59] and gelatinases were fractionated and identified on zymography by gelatin-SDS-PAGE [85]. After Coomassie Blue R250 staining, excess stain was removed to visualize gelatinases as clear unstained or less stained bands. Semiquatification of gelatinase(s) bands was performed by densitometry.

Levels of TGF-B$_1$ secreted iInto RCM by retinal explants

PN2 and PN7 *wt* and *rdl* mice pups were decapitated; retinas with attached RPE were dissected from the enucleated eyes and cultured for 26 and 21 days, respectively in serum free R-16 complete medium containing bovine serum albumin (BSA) [21]. RCM samples were collected on alternate days, stored at -20°C until analyzed and R-16 complete medium was replenished. After activation, TGF-β$_1$ and TGF-β$_2$ secreted into the RCM were quantified by ELISA as per protocols provided by the manufacturer (RandD Systems Quantikine Kits each specific for TGF-β$_1$ and TGF-β$_2$) using ELISA plate reader (Molecular Devices Corporation, USA) at 450 nm with λ correction at 545 nm. Since TGF-β$_1$ and TGF-β$_2$ were measured after activation so the results reported here do not distinguish between the active and latent forms of TGF-β$_1$ and TGF-β$_2$.

Antioxidant Treatments in In Vitro and In Vivo [See Reference 96 For Procedures]

For *in vitro* studies PN5 retinas were cultured until the *in vitro* age of PN18 in the presence of antioxidants. The antioxidants GSH (10 μg / ml), α-lipoic acid (10 µg / ml), zeaxanthin (0.67 µg / ml) and lutein (0.67 µg / ml) were provided individually or all four were combined and added to the R-16 complete culture medium. For *in vivo* studies PN3 *rd1* pups were administered GSH (10 mg / kg body weight), α-lipoic acid (10 mg / kg body weight), zeaxanthin (0.67 mg / kg body weight), and lutein (0.67 / kg body weight) individually or in combination by oral route until the age of PN10 or PN16. The calculated volume of dissolved and diluted antioxidants to be fed was increased with the increase in body weight measured on alternate days. Control *rd1* mice received the vehicle alone. Retinas were dissected and those from *in vitro* and *in vivo* treatments were evaluated for histological changes and DNA oxidation [96].

Statistical Analyses [See References 6, 7 and 9 For Levels of Significance]

Statistical analysis was by one-way analysis of variance and Fisher's protected least significant differences post hoc comparisons (StatView Software, SAS, Chicago; IL, USA).

Results

The Rd1 Retina Showed Less Sialylation of Sgag at PN2/PN7 and Lower Proteins with Higher Sgag at PN21 and PN28

PN2 and PN7 *wt* extracts showed higher extent of sialylation of sGAG component of proteoglycans as compared to *rd1* extracts, whereas PN14 *rd1* extracts displayed an opposite relationship; PN7 and PN14 *rd1* extracts showed higher galactosylation of proteoglycans as compared to *wt* extracts and PN21, PN28 *wt* proteoglycans also showed higher extent of sialylation [Figure 3 E, F, G and H]. Thus there was delayed sialylation or premature desialylation in *rd1* retina. The protein content in *wt* and *rd1* retinal extract was respectively increased and decreased while the reverse was the case for sGAG content [Figure 4]. In addition, PN14, -21 and -28 *rd1* retinal extracts showed an accumulation of sulfate rich sGAG with loss of core proteins of proteoglycans [reference 6 Figure 7 A, B, C, and D].

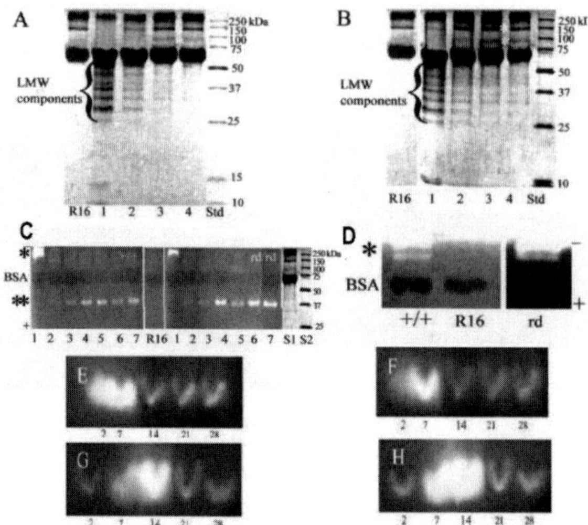

Figure 3. SDS-PAGE and zymography of RCM shows gelatinases: Unlike the SDS-PAGE profile of R16 complete medium, the retinal conditioned medium (RCM) collected on div (days in vitro in culture) -3 (lane 1), -5 (lane 2), -8 (lane 3), -10 (lane 4) from PN7 wt (A) and rd1 (B) retinal explants show presence of decreasing extent of low molecular weight (LMW) proteins. In case of RCM from wt explants such protein bands disappear after div 5 (A, lane 3) but persist in that from rd1 explants (B). Since molecular weight of protein bands in RCM are lower than that of those present in R16 medium so these bands possibly represent secreted proteins including proteinases and degradation products of retinal proteins, BSA and BSA associated globulins added to the R16 medium.Gelatin-SDS-PAGE zymography of RCM from PN2 (D) and PN7 (C) wt and rd1 retinal explants initially showed high molecular weight (* , HMW) secreted gelatinases (broad white bands near the origin) or their oligomer(s) and / or complexes with substrates / inhibitors. Secretion of HMW gelatinases by PN7 explants was extremely decreased in subsequent collections of RCM and changed over to low molecular weight gelatinases [** , LMW white bands showed increased intensity as the culture period was increased through div -2-3♦ (lane 1), -5 (lane 2), -7 (lane 3), -9-10♦ (lane4), -12 (lane5), -16-14♦ (lane 6), -20-17♦ (lane 7)]. The LMW gelatinases possibly represent stromelysin or MMP-7 or MMP-13 or MMP-14 which activate inactive zymogen forms of MMP-2 and MMP-9 and also degrade extracellular matrix constituents. ♦ div for some rd1 explants and others are for wt, wt as well as rd1 explants. Lectin blotting (E, F, G and H) showed that PN2 and PN7 wt extracts (E) as compared to rd1 extracts (G) had higher extent of sialylation of proteoglycans as observed by wheat germ agglutinin reaction and reverse was the case for PN14 rd1 extracts; PN7 and PN14 rd1 extracts (H) as compared to wt extracts (F) showed higher galactosylation of proteoglycans by peanut agglutinin reaction; and PN21, PN28 wt extract proteoglycans also showed higher extent of sialylation. Proteoglycans in the neonatal rd1 extracts were either desialylated or their sialylation was delayed.
Copyright Permission Reference 6

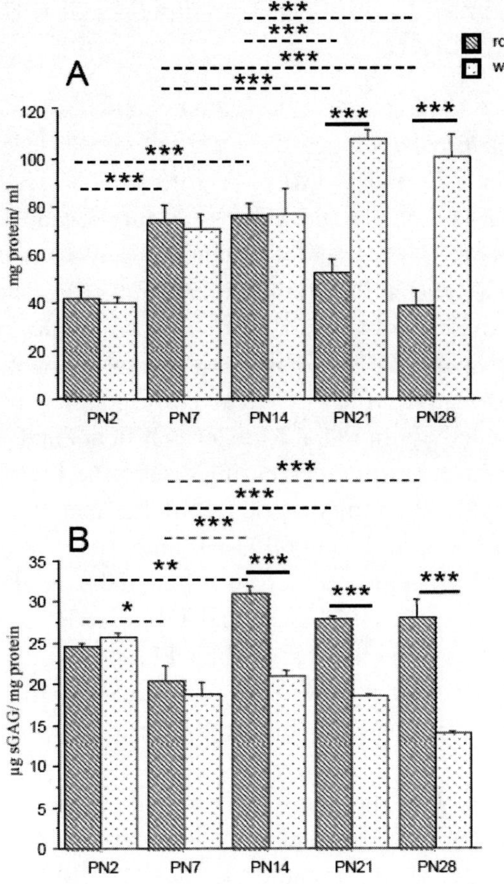

Figure 4. Developmental and comparative changes in the levels of total proteins (A) and sGAG (B) in the wt and rd1 retinal extracts:During the PN2, -7 and -14 stages, when the retina is developing, the total protein content in wt and rd1 retinal extracts was increased and this continued during PN21 and PN28 stages of wt retina but in rd1 retina which undergoes degeneration during this period, the protein content was decreased. Except for PN2 stage, the level of total sGAG in rd1 retinal extracts was higher than that in wt extracts. During the development of retina at PN2 and PN7 stage of both genotypes, the level of sGAG was relatively lower and remained unchanged in wt retina but was increased in rd1 retina which was undergoing degeneration. The significance of differences was in the range of *P<0.05, **P<0.01 and ***P<0.001. Differences within rd1 (dashed lines), and between wt and rd1 (solid lines) have been marked in horizontal direction. Copyright Permission Reference 6.

Cellular Sources and Levels of Proteinases and their Endogenous Inhibitors

Identification of retinal cell sources of proteinases and their endogenous inhibitors

In PN2 *wt* and *rd1* retinas MMP-2 [Figure 5, lane 1, *rd1*- A, B, C, D and E, lane 2, *wt*- F, G, H, I and J] and MMP-9 [Figure 5, lane 3, *rd1*- K, L, M, N and O, lane 4, *wt*- P, Q, R, S and T] immunoreactivity was observed in the subretinal space, whereas in PN7 retinas it was in the IPL and OPL of both the *wt* and *rd1* retinas. PN14, -21 and -28 *wt* retinas showed MMP-2 immunoreactivity in the OPL and inner segments of photoreceptors, in the interphotoreceptor matrix (IPM); whereas corresponding *rd1* retinas showed MMP-2 immunoreactivity in radial Mueller cell fibers and in the diminishing subretinal space and it was in a decreasing order. The PN14, -21 and -28 *rd1* retinas showed MMP-9 immunreaction in OPL and collapsing subretinal space, whereas *wt* retinas did so in OPL and inner segment of IPM [Figure 5]. Both in PN2 *wt* and *rd1* retinas cathepsin B immunoreactivity was observed in the RPE, subretinal space, IPL, ILM and GCL; at PN7 stage cathepsin B immunoreactivity was also observed in the OPL and INL. At PN14, -21 and -28 stages *wt* and *rd1* retinas showed immunoreactivity in the RPE, INL and GCL but not in the OPL and ILM [Figure 6, lane 3, *wt*- A, B, C, D and E, lane 4, *rd1*- F, G, H, I and J].

Both PN2 and PN7 *wt* and *rd1* retinal sections showed TIMP-1 immunoreactivity in OPL and subretinal space; PN14, -21 and -28 *rd1* sections showed petechial immunoreactions for TIMP-1 in collapsing subretinal space, whereas corresponding *wt* retinal sections showed weak TIMP-1 immunoreactivity in inner segments of the enlarging subretinal space and clear intense immunoreactivity at the base of the IPM [Figure 7, lane 1, *rd1*- A, B, C, D and E, lane 2, *wt*- F, G, H, I and J]. At PN2, TIMP-2 immunoreactivity was present in the subretinal space; at PN7 maximum immunoreactivity accumulated in IPM both of *rd1* and *wt* retinas, more so in the latter. PN14, -21 and -28 *wt* retinas showed TIMP-2 immunoreactivity in the OPL and inner segments of photoreceptors in the IPM, whereas corresponding *rd1* retinas showed decreasing TIMP-2 immunoreactivity in radial Mueller cell fibers and the diminishing subretinal space [Figure 7, lane 3, *rd1*- K, L, M, N and O, lane 4 *wt*- P, Q, R, S and T]. Optic nerve head and RGC showed cystatin C immunoreactivity [Figure 6, lane 5, B, C]. PN2 *wt* and *rd1* retinal sections showed cystatin C immunoreactivity in RPE, GCL

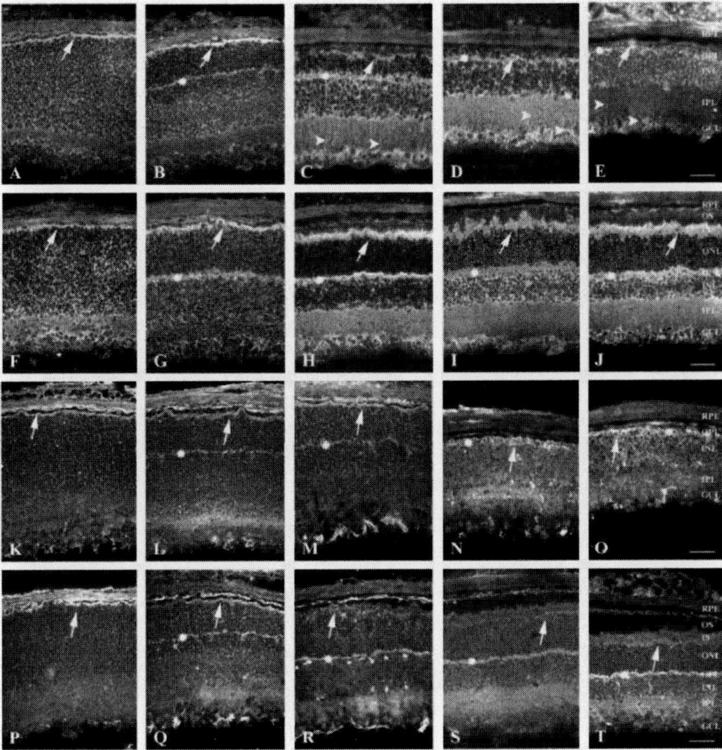

Figure 5. Developmental cellular immunolocalization of MMP-2 (lane 1, A-E rd1 and lane 2, F-J wt) and MMP-9 (lane 3, K-O rd1 and lane 4, P-T wt) in immersion fixed retinas: Lanes 1, -2: The developing subretinal space in PN2 retina of both genotypes showed MMP-2 (arrows A, F). At PN7, the MMP-2 labeling accumulated in the IPM (arrows B, G) and also appeared in the OPL (stars B, G) of wt and rd1 retinas. Subsequently PN14 (C, H), -21 (D, I) and -28 (E, J) rd1 photoreceptors degenerate and MMP-2 labeling was observed in the subretinal space and in radial Mueller cell fibers (arrow heads) of rd1 retinas and it diminished with the progress of degeneration. In PN14, -21 and -28 wt retinas the MMP-2 reaction was unchanged (H, I, and J) and was limited to the inner part of IPM (arrow H).Lanes 3, -4: The developing and expanding subretinal space of PN2 (arrows K, P) retina and OPL of PN7 (stars L, Q) retina of both genotypes showed MMP-9 immunolabeling. The MMP-9 immunolabeling of the subretinal space of PN14, -21 and -28 rd1 retinas (arrows M, N and O) was persistent. MMP-9 immunolabeling in the OPL was also persistent at all the remaining time points both in wt (Q, R, S and T) and rd1 (L, M, N and O) retinas. Unlike MMP-2 labeling, MMP-9 labeling was lacking in the radial Mueller cell fibers of rd1 retinas. In wt retina (arrows R, S and T) MMP-9 labeling of IPM decreased as it matured. RPE, retinal pigmented epithelium; IS, OS, inner- and outer photoreceptor segments; IPL, OPL, inner- and outer plexiform layers; INL, ONL, inner- and outer nuclear layers; GCL, ganglion cell layer; IPM, interphotoreceptor matrix. Scale bar = 50 μm.
Copyright Permission Reference 6

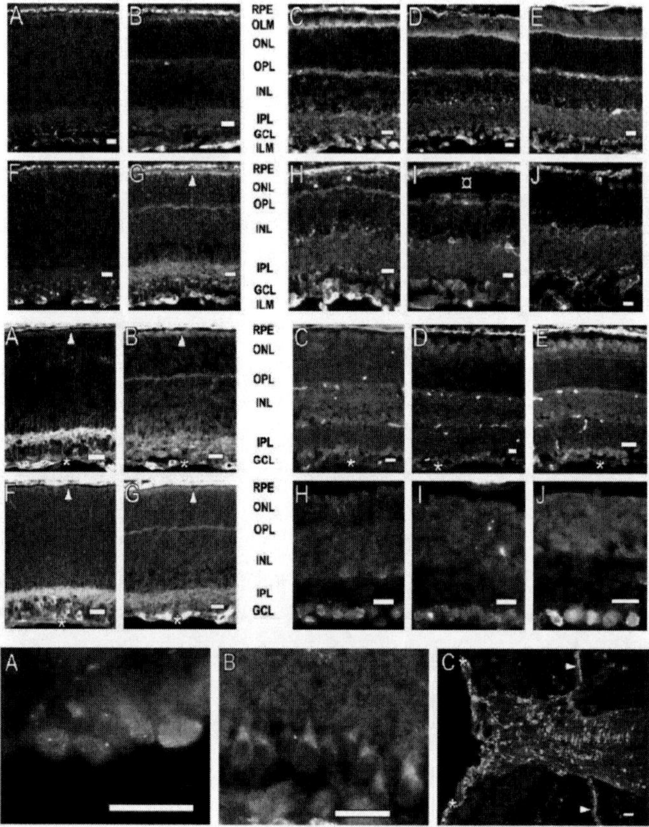

Figure 6. Developmental cellular immunolocalization of cystatin C (lane 1, A-E wt and lane 2, F-J rd1) and cathepsin B (lane 3, A-E wt and lane 4, F-J rd1) in immersion fixed retinas: Lanes 1, -2: The retinas at PN2 showed cystatin C labeling in RPE GCL, and ILM; at PN7 (wt - B and rd1 - F) cystatin C labeling was also observed in OLM (arrowhead) and OPL (B). PN2 and PN7 rd1 retinas (F, G) showed similar localization of cystatin C. At PN14, -21 and -28 (C, D, E) in wt retinas increasing cystatin C labeling was observed in RPE, OLM, inner retina, GCL and ILM, whereas corresponding rd1 retinas (H, I, J) showed relatively stronger cystatin C labeling in the RPE, INL, GCL and ILM.Lanes 3, -4: The wt (A) and rd1 (F) retinas at PN2 showed cathepsin B labeling in RPE, subretinal space (arrowhead), IPL, ILM (*) and GCL (A); at PN7 wt (B) and rd1 (G) showed cathepsin B labeling additionally in the OPL and INL (cathepsin B labeling in the IPL and GCL of PN2 and PN7 retinas of both genotypes suggested synaptogenesis and PCD of RGC); PN14, -21 and -28, the wt (C, D and E) and rd1 (H, I, J) retinas showed cathepsin B labeling in the RPE, INL and GCL but not in the OPL and ILM, wt retinas additionally showed cathepsin B labeling of capillaries suggesting that the vasculature are also a source of cathepsin B. This implied that retinal cells in wt retinas by themselves produced much less cathepsin B. Copyright Permission Reference 7. Immunostaining of optic nerve head for cathepsin B

(lane 5, PN21 rd1, A) and cystatin C (lane 5, PN14 rd1, B and C): Lanes 5: Petechial labeling of cathepsin B in RGC (A) of both genotypes suggested its vesicular localization in the cytoplasm. Higher cathepsin B may be involved in PCD of RGC of PN2 and PN7 retinas of both genotypes but during degeneration in PN14, -21 and -28 rd1 retinas it may induce the RGC to activate microglia cells. Faint peripheral and strong polar axonal localization of cystatin C (B, enlargement from lane 4 H) suggested that cystatin C was also localized in the cytoplasm and was in the direction of the axonal transport. This is apparent from the low magnification image of optic nerve head (C). The extensively cystatin C labeled structures situated perpendicular to the direction of the optic nerve head (C) may also represent astrocytes and oligodendrcyte glial cells surrounding the optic nerve axons. The extensive cystatin C label diminished in a descending order from the optic nerve head in the intraocular through intraorbital segments of the optic nerve and suggested dispersion of cystatin C along the optic nerve. RPE, retinal pigmented epithelium; OLM, ILM, outer- and inner limiting membranes; ONL, INL, outer and inner nuclear layers; OPL, IPL,.

and ILM and PN7 retinal sections of both genotypes showed additional immunoreactivity in OLM and OPL. At PN14, -21 and -28 cystatin C immunoreactivity was observed in RPE, INL, GCL and ILM of both genotypes [Figure 6, lane 1, *wt*- A, B, C, D and E, lane 2, *rd1*- F, G, H, I and J]. The immunoreactivity for TIMP-1, TIMP-2 and cystatin C, endogenous inhibitors of MMPs and cathepsins, respectively was more intense in different regions of PN14, -21 and -28 *wt* retinal sections than in the corresponding *rd1* sections.

Proteinases were shown in RCM of both genotypes by SDS-PAGE and zymography

The R-16 complete medium contains BSA, and consequently showed bands of BSA and BSA associated globulin by SDS-PAGE analyses [Figure 3 A, B]. However, similar analyses of RCM collected at different times of culture showed distinct low molecular weight (LMW) components which were not present in the R-16 complete medium. The origin of the LMW components was possibly the proteins secreted by retinal explants and degradation products originating from proteins of the retinal explants and BSA and BSA associated globulins from the R-16 complete medium.

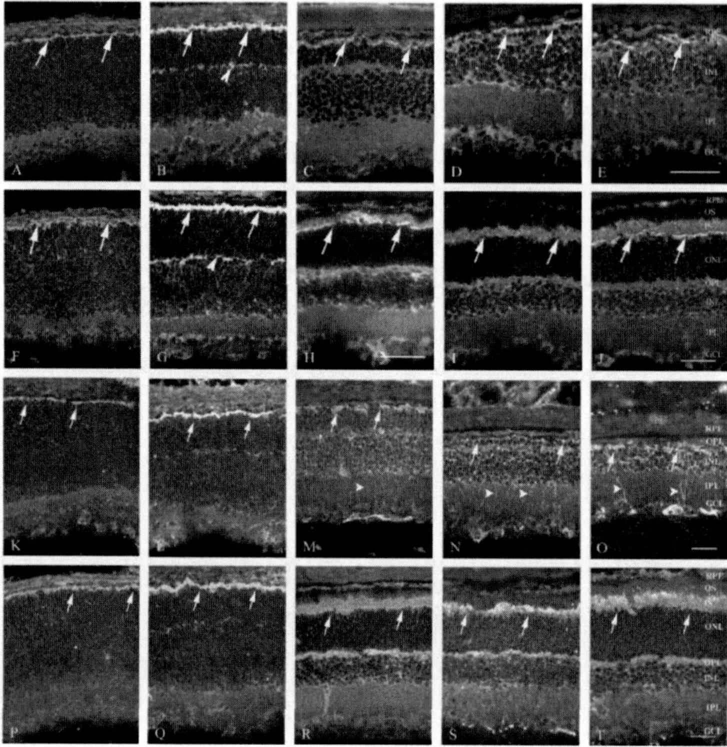

Figure 7. Developmental cellular immunolocalization of TIMP-1 (lane 1, A-E rd1 and lane 2, F-J wt) and TIMP-2 (lane 3, K-O rd1 and lane 4, P-T wt) in immersion fixed retinas: Lanes 1, -2: Subretinal space (arrows) in PN2 and PN7 wt (F, G) and rd1 (A, B) retinas showed TIMP-1 immunolabeling which was also evident in the OPL (arrowheads) of PN7 retinas of both genotypes (G, B). The PN14, -21 and -28 rd1 retinas showed weaker immunolabeling for TIMP-1 in the degenerating subretinal space (arrows, C, D and E) whereas in corresponding wt retinas the expanding subretinal space shows a weak TIMP-1 immunolabeling which was intense in the base of the IPM (arrows, H, I and J). The retinal distribution of TIMP-1 corresponds to that of MMP-9 in the two genotypes, respectively.Lanes 3, -4: Subretinal space (arrows) in PN2 and PN7 wt (P, Q) and rd1 (K, L) retinas showed TIMP-2 immunolabeling. PN14, -21 and -28 rd1 retinas showed immunolabeling for TIMP-2 in the IPM, OPL(arrows M, N and O) and radial Mueller cell fibers (arrowheads M, N and O), whereas in corresponding wt retinas the TIMP-2 immunolabeling was limited to the inner segment of the IPM and OPL (arrows, R, S and T). The retinal distribution of TIMP-2 corresponded to that of MMP-2 in the two genotypes respectively. RPE, retinal pigmented epithelium; IS, OS, inner- and outer photoreceptor segments; IPL, OPL, inner- and outer plexiform layers; INL, ONL, inner- and outer nuclear layers; GCL, ganglion cell layer; IPM, interphotoreceptor matrix. Scale bar = 50 μm. Copyright Permission Reference 6

Gelatin zymography of RCM collected at different times of culture of PN7 *wt* and *rd1* retinal explants initially showed intense bands of high molecular weight [* Figure 3 C] gelatinases. These were faintly visible during prolongation of the culture period. RCM collected after such prolonged cultivation showed a major LMW gelatinase band [** Figure 3 C] which could possibly represent MMP-14 as indicated by the molecular weight. Gelatin zymography of RCM collected at different times of culture of PN2 *wt* and *rd1* retinal explants showed gelatinases of higher molecular weight [Figure 3 D] only during the first collection of RCM while RCM collected on prolonged cultivation lacked gelatinases. Possibly the level of LMW gelatinases in RCM from PN2 explants was too low for clear detection by zymography. Fluorometric quantification of proteinases secreted by PN2 [Figure 8 A] and PN7 [Figure 8 B] *wt* and *rd1* explants into RCM for up to PN28 days in culture showed that proteinases and gelatinases secreted by PN2 explants of both genotypes were not detectable after prolonged culture. However, higher levels of proteinases and gelatinases were secreted by PN7 *rd1* explants after prolonged culture *in vitro* [Figure 8 D]. Secretion of gelatinases by PN7 *wt* and *rd1* explants was similar up to div7 and thereafter it was higher by *rd1* explants [Figure 8 C, D].

The Rd1 Retina Showed Imbalance in Proteinases and their Inhibitors

MMP-2 [Figure 9 A] and MMP-9 [Figure 9 B] activities in *wt* retinal extracts decreased with age from PN2 to PN28. PN2 *rd1* extract had higher activities of MMP-2 and MMP-9 and after that MMP-2 activity remained constant but higher than those in corresponding *wt* extracts, whereas MMP-9 activity by contrast increased with age. Total cathepsin [reference 9 Figure 2], cathepsin B, -S and –L [Figure 10 A, B and C] activities in *wt* extracts at different stages were unchanged but lower than those in corresponding *rd1* extracts. Activities of cathepsins in the *rd1* extracts increased with age. Cathepsin S activity in PN2 *wt* extracts was significantly higher but that in *rd1* extracts nonsignificantly increased with age. PN2 *wt* extract had highest cathepsin S activity.

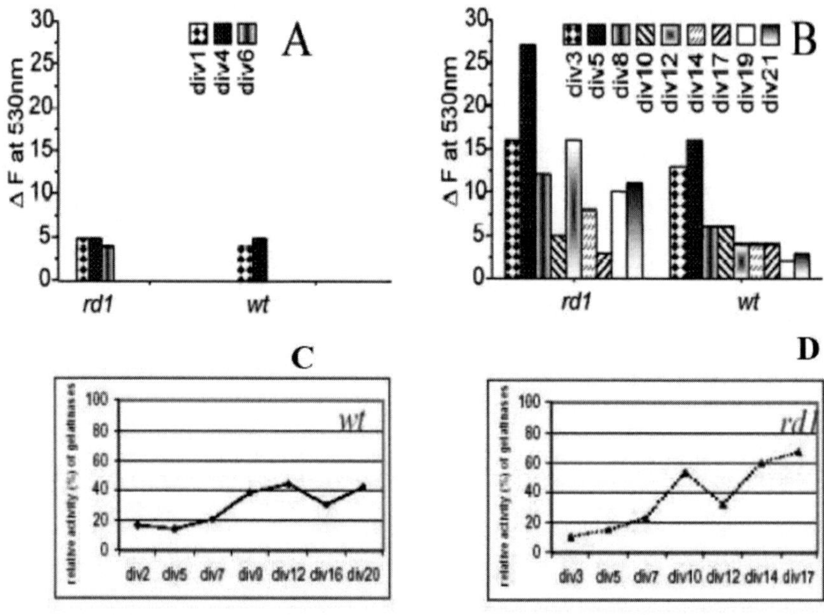

Figure 8. Fluorometry and densitometry of zymographs of RCM from PN7 rd1 retinal explants showed higher secretion of proteinases and gelatinases: Fluorometric quantification of proteinases secreted by PN2 (A) and PN7 (B) wt and rd1 retinal explants into RCM for up to PN28 days in vitro culture (div) showed that proteinases (A, B) and gelatinases (C, D) secreted by PN2 explants of both genotypes were not detectable after prolonged culture. However, higher levels of proteinases and gelatinases were secreted by PN7 rd1 explants after prolonged culture in vitro. Secretion of gelatinases by PN7 wt and rd1 explants was similar up to div7 and thereafter it was higher by rd1 explants (C, D). Copyright Permission Reference 6,7

TIMP-1 levels in *wt* retinal extracts decreased with age, whereas those of *rd1* extracts increased with age from PN7 stage onwards. PN2 *rd1* and *wt* extracts had high and similar levels of TIMP-1 [Figures 9 D] and TIMP-2 [Figures 9 B] than those in retinal extracts from other stages of development. TIMP-2 in *rd1* extracts decreased up to PN14 and then increased again up to PN28. In PN2 and PN7 *wt* extracts TIMP-2 level was similar but was decreased after that. At all stages, cystatin C level in *rd1* extracts were higher than that in corresponding *wt* extracts. In *wt* extracts cystatin C increased up to PN14 and then decreased but was higher than that in PN2 extracts [Figure 10 D].

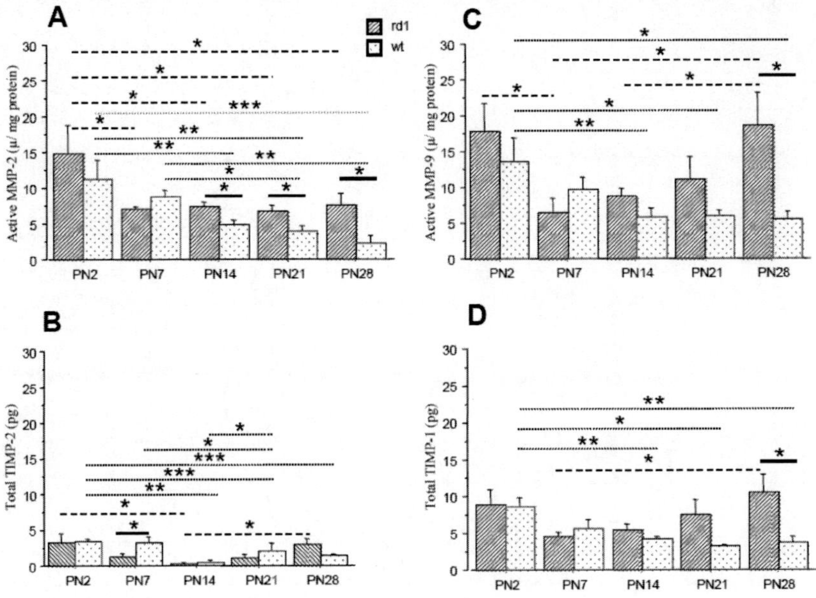

Figure 9. Developmental and comparative changes in the levels of active MMP-2 (A), TIMP-2 (B) active MMP-9 (C) and TIMP-1 (D) in the *wt* and *rd1* retinal extracts: At all time points except PN7, the activity of MMP-2 was higher in *rd1* retinal extracts (A). Both in *wt* and *rd1* the MMP-2 activity was highest at PN2 and declined with the development of *wt* retina but in *rd1* retina the MMP-9 activity decreases at PN7 and remained unchanged thereafter. At all time points except PN7, the activity of MMP-9 was higher in *rd1* retinal extracts (C). In the *wt* retina the MMP-9 activity was highest at PN2 and thereafter it declined with the development of retina. Whereas, in *rd1* retina it declined at PN7 and thereafter, the MMP-9 activity increased to the initial level (C) and suggested that relative to MMP-2 activity, the MMP-9 activity was related more to the degenerative process in *rd1* retina. At all time points the level of TIMP-2 (B) was lower than that of TIMP-1 (D). In *rd1* the level of TIMP-2 decreased to a minimum at PN14 and then increased to the initial level, whereas the level of TIMP-2 in PN2 and PN7 *wt* extracts was similar and higher than that in *rd1* extracts and the subsequent increase was lower that in *rd1* extracts. At all time points except PN7, the level of TIMP-1 was higher in *rd1* retinal extracts (D). In the *wt* retina the TIMP-1 level was highest at PN2 and thereafter it declined with the development of retina. Whereas, in *rd1* retina it declined at PN7 and thereafter, the TIMP-1 level increased more than the initial level (D) and in spite this increase in the level of TIMP-1, the activity of MMP-9 was higher and could not prevent the degeneration of retina. The significance of differences was in the range of *P<0.05, **P<0.01 and ***P<0.001. Differences within *wt* (dotted lines), within *rd1* (dashed lines), and between *wt* and *rd1* (solid lines) have been marked in horizontal direction *Copyright Permission Reference 6.*

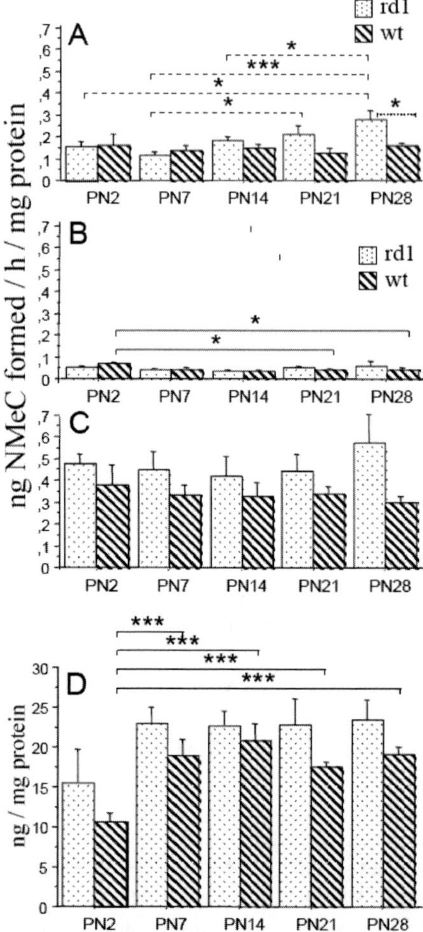

Figure 10. Developmental and comparative changes in the levels of cysteine cathepsin B (A), cathepsin S (B), cathepsin L(C) and cystatin C (D) in the wt and rd1 retinal extracts: Cysteine cathepsin B, cathepsin S and cathepsin L (increased from PN14 onwards) activity increased with age in rd1 but remained unchanged and lower in wt (being highest at PN2) retinal extracts. Irrespective of the protein content cathepsin activities were higher in rd1 extracts. The proportion of cathepsin activities decreased in the following descending order: cathepsin L< cathepsin B < cathepsin S. In spite of higher cystatin C level, the cathepsin activities in rd1 extracts were higher than those in wt extracts. After PN14 stage cystatin C level in wt extracts declined, whereas that in rd1 extracts remained unchanged. The significance of differences was in the range of *P<0.05, **P<0.01 and ***P<0.001. Differences within wt (solid brackets), within rd1 (dashed brackets), and between wt and rd1 (dotted brackets) have been marked in horizontal direction. *Copyright Permission Reference 7*

At PN2 there was no difference between the genotypes in the retinal levels of TIMP-1 and TIMP-2 but in *rd1* extracts of all stages cystatin C content was higher. At PN7 stage TIMP-1, TIMP-2 and cystatin C levels were higher in *wt* extracts and in PN14, -21 and -28 *rd1* extracts TIMP-1 and cystatin C contents were higher [Figure 8 D and Figure 10 D]. In spite of the increase in the levels of inhibitors, the activities of proteinases were still higher.

Secretion of proteinases by Rd1 explants was higher but with less of TGF-B$_1$

PN2 *wt* and *rd1* explants secreted lower levels of TGF β_1 as compared to PN7 *wt* and *rd1* explants. TGF-β_1 level in RCM from PN2 *rd1* retinal explants cultured for 5 to -12 days *in vitro* (div) and those from PN7 *rd1* cultured for div 1 to -5 were too low to be measured by the ELISA method used or TGF-β_1 was degraded by increased proteinases. However, PN2 and PN7 *wt* retinal explants secreted TGF-β_1 into RCM throughout the period of culture and its level was higher than that secreted by corresponding *rd1* explants (Table 1). TGF-β_2 was not detectable in any of the RCM samples from PN2 / PN7 *wt* and *rd1* retinal explants and the ELISA kits used during the study were, therefore, not sensitive enough for the purpose.

The level of total proteinases in RCM collected for 12 div from PN7 *rd1* retinal explants was significantly (P<0.05) higher than that by corresponding PN7 *wt* explants. Levels of active and total MMP-9, TIMP-1 and ratio of TIMP-1 to active MMP-2 in RCM collected for 12 div from PN7 *rd1* explants was higher and ratio of TIMP-1 to active MMP-9 and total MMP-2 was lower than that by corresponding PN7 *wt* explants (Table 2) suggesting that the secretion of proteinase activity by *rd1* retina was higher. PN2 explants of both genotypes had limited capacity to secrete cystatin C and cathepsins which decreased to undetectable levels after 6 days in culture (data not shown). As compared to PN7 *wt* explants, PN7 *rd1* explants secreted higher levels of both cystatin C and active cathepsins into the RCM collected during the period of 21 days and the last 11 days in culture. In spite of higher secretion of cathepsin and its inhibitor cystatin C, the ratio of active cathepsins to cystatin C was still higher and represented higher cathepsin activities and degenerative changes in the *rd1* retina (Table 3).

GST or a Combination of Antioxidants Rescued Rod Photoreceptors from Rd1 Retina Showing Oxidative Stress

Both α-GST and μ-GST levels showed a peak at PN7 in *wt* and *rd1* extracts and thereafter these were lower in *rd1* retinas [reference 8 Figure 1 B, D]. In *wt* retinal extracts GPx and GSH decreased with age from PN2 to PN21; whereas in PN2 *rd1* GSH and malondialdehyde levels were higher than that in *wt* extracts and GPx as well as GR activities increased with age and malondialdehyde decreased from PN2 to PN14 *rd1* extracts [reference 9 Figure 1 A, B, C and D]. An increase in malondialdehyde and a decrease in GST levels in PN2 *rd1* retina indicated an oxidative stress early during the postnatal development. Thus in *rd1* and *wt* retinas higher oxidative stress was observed at early / late and late stages of development, respectively.

Histological analysis of the *rd1* retina demonstrated oxidative DNA damage as revealed by the presence of 8-hydroxy deoxyguanosine, an oxidized purine base in DNA. The *rd1* but not *wt* retinas showed presence of 8-hydroxy deoxyguanosine in DNA of the cells of ONL [reference 96 Figure 1 A, B, C, D, E and F]. These changes in PN11 *rd1* retinas were partially reversed after feeding of a combination of all four antioxidants namely lutein, zeaxanthin, GSH, and α-lipoic acid from PN3 stage onwards [reference 96 Figure 3, A, B, C, D, E and F]. The number of photoreceptor rows in *rd1* retinas was higher, both under *in vitro* and *in vivo* treatments with the above referred combination of antioxidants [reference 96 Figure 2 A, B, C and D; and Figure 4 A, B, C, D and E].

Table1. Secretion of TGF-β1 (pg/ml/day, Mean ± SE) into the retinal conditioned medium (RCM) by PN2 and PN7 *wt* and *rd1* retinal explants cultured for 12 days in vitro (div)

	wt	*rd1*
PN2	19.3 ± 5.3	9.1 ± 6.6[¶]
PN7	41.3 ± 6.9*	14.0 ± 6.1[æ]

* RCM from PN7 wt retinas has significantly higher (at 5% level) TGF-β1 values (pooled data) than those in RCM from PN2 wt and rd1 and PN7 rd1 retinas cultured in vitro. TGF-β1 level in RCM from PN2 rd1 retinas cultured for div 5 to -12 (¶) and those from PN7 rd1 cultured for div 1 to -5 (æ) were too low to be measured by the method used. The method used could not detect TGF-β2 levels in any of the RCM samples.

Table 2. Secretion of MMPs and TIMPs (Mean ± SE) into the conditioned medium (RCM) by PN7 *wt* and *rd1* retinal explants cultured for 12 days in vitro (div).

	wt	*rd1*
Total Proteinases (div 10 to -21)	3.83 ±0.54	8.83 ± 1.89*
Active MMP-9¥	1.09 ± 0.11	1.34 ± 0.05¶
Total MMP-9¥	2.59 ± 0.04	2.83 ± 0.08¶
Active MMP-2¥	3.25 ± 0.10	3.08 ± 0.12§
Total MMP-2¥	23.8 ± 2.9	30.8 ± 5.0§
TIMP-1Л	4.08 ± 0.19	4.66 ± 0.65§
TIMP-2 Л	0.30 ± 0.03	0.31 ± 0.03NS
Ratio of TIMP-1 to:		
Active MMP-9	3.81 ± 0.31	3.51 ± 0.58NS
Total MMP-9	1.57 ± 0.05	1.66 ± 0.27NS
Active MMP-2	1.26 ± 0.06	1.51 ± 0.22§
Total MMP-2	0.18 ± 0.02	0.15 ± 0.01§

RCM was collected on alternate days, analyzed and data from div 7 to -12 RCM was pooled. The period of culture includes the development of *wt* retina and progression of degeneration of *rd1* retina. Proteinases (F Δ at 530 nm / 100 µl of RCM); * p-value significant at 5% level; [¶] p-value (0.10, 0.06) close to significance at 5% level; [§] non-significant but the p-values are low and / or the differences between the means are large; [NS] non-significant; [Л] ng/ml RCM/day; [¥] ΔAU at 405 nm /h^2*10^3 in RCM. RCM shows imbalance in MMPs and TIMPs axis, in favor of MMPs.

Table 3. Comparative secretion of cysteine proteinases and cystatin C (Mean ± SE) by PN7 *wt* and *rd1* retinal explants into the retinal conditioned medium (RCM) during 21 days of culture.

	wt	rd1
Cysteine protinases§ (ΔF/100 µl RCM)	6.44 ± 1.60 (33.0)	12.00 ± 2.38 (46.7)
Cysteine protinases¶ (ΔF/100 µl RCM)	3.83 ± 0.54 (19.6)	8.83 ± 1.89 (34.4)
Cystatin C (µg/ml RCM/day)	0.195 ± 0.03	0.257 ± 0.06

[§] represents analyses of RCM collected during all the 21 days of culture,

[¶] represents analyses of RCM collected during the last 11 days of culture.

The values in parentheses represent ratio of active cathepsins to their endogenous inhibitor cystatin C and indicate that in spite of higher secretion of cystatin C the RCM from *rd1* explants have relatively higher levels of cathepsins which contribute to the degenerative changes in *rd1* retina.

Discussion

This chapter reports the levels of TGF-β_1, sialylation of proteoglycans, proteinases and their inhibitors and the cellular sources of proteinases and their inhibitors in retina of *rd1* mouse model of retinitis pigmentosa relative to the *wt* control. The retina of the *rd1* mouse shows degeneration of rod photoreceptors with the reorganization of neural and vascular networks, swelling of mitochondria, imbalance in proteinases and deficiency of vasculature. Some of these changes are observed even during retinal cell differentiation and photoreceptor development [2, 6, 7, 39 and 95]. Malfunctioning mitochondria not only decrease the production of ATP and increase the leakage of ROS and Ca^{2+} ions but can also inhibit the axonal transport processes and lead to defective synaptogenesis [35]. Although controversy exists about the *in vivo* regulation of calpain activity, yet it is accepted that oxidative stress induced oxidation of proteins and unsaturated fatty acids in the plasma membranes and cell organelle membranes increases cytosolic Ca^{2+} ions level, with the possible concomitant activation of calpain [77]. As soon as cytosolic Ca^{2+} ions return to physiological levels, the calpain activity reverts to normal [77]. Moreover, calpain activity is regulated by the levels of its endogenous inhibitor calpastatin and any decrease in its level would increase calpain activity [86, 87]. Activation of calpain affects membranes of cell organelles and releases lysosomal enzymes including cysteine cathepsins. Release of Ca^{2+} ions from the mitochondria, Golgi apparatus (GA) and endoplasmic reticulum (ER) due to PDE mutation and increased ROS in *rd1* retina possibly increased the calpain activity [86] and also released lysosomal cathepsins. Distict proteinase families like caspases and calpains cleave plasma membrane Ca^{2+} ATPases and Na^+/Ca^{2+} ion exchangers and possibly other ion exchangers and create intracellular accumulation of Ca^{2+} ions and neuronal death [125, 126, 127, 128 and 129]. This in turn would maintain a vicious cycle of damage to the organization of plasma membranes and cell organelles followed by release of cathepsins, Ca^{2+} ions and ROS. The involvement of MMPs, serine proteinases and cysteine cathepsins B, -L, and -S in development, remodeling of ECM for angiogenesis and degeneration of different tissues has been reported [16, 40, 56, 64, 104 and 116]. Therefore, the present studies on histochemical and biochemical changes partially elucidate some of the mechanisms of pathogenesis of inherited retinal degeneration like retinitis pigmentosa.

Mueller Cells were the Additional Source of Proteinases in Rd1 Retina

Retinal cells form a network and are generally described as being organized into different layers. Development, remodeling and tissue destruction under physiological conditions and during neurodegenerative, vascular, inflammatory diseases and tumor progression is dependent on the duration and balance between the activities of proteinases namely MMPs, serine proteinase plasminogen activators (uPA, tPA), cysteine proteinases (calpain and cathepsins) and their respective endogenous inhibitors TIMPs, PAI-1, calpastatin, and cystatin C [6, 7, 24, 28, 80, 100, 104, 105 and 117]. The combined proteinase activities of retinal resident and inflammatory cells as well as vasculature are the likely sources of these proteinases and their inhibitors.

The main source of MMP-9 and MMP-2 in the mouse retina is the RPE [3] but during the present studies MMPs and TIMPs immunoreaction was observed in the IPM but not in the RPE. This anomaly may be due to their secretion into the IPM by the RPE. MMP-2, MMP-9, TIMP-1, cathepsin B and cystatin C were observed in the subretinal space of PN2 *wt* and *rd1* retinas and in the OPL and IPL at PN7 stage which pointed to the photoreceptors and integrator neurons as the source of these enzymes. Detection of cathepsin B and cystatin C in GCL and ILM at PN2 stage of *wt* and *rd1* retina suggested that RGC and Mueller cell end feet processes were also the source of this proteolytic system. Subsequent observation of cathepsin B in the OPL and INL and of cystatin C in the OLM and OPL in PN7 retinas of both genotypes indicated that photoreceptors and their processes expressed cathepsin B, whereas cystatin C was expressed by photoreceptors, integrator neurons and Mueller cells. The results are compatible with the suggestion that increased proteinases generate paths in extracellular matrix for the extension and branching of neuronal and vascular processes and for the lay out of new matrix during the postnatal development of retina. MMP-2 and TIMP-2 immunopattern were similar in *wt* and *rd1* mice and their initially increased expression by Mueller cells in *rd1* was followed by a relative decrease during *rd1* retinal degeneration. IPM showed higher intensity of immunoreaction for MMP-2 and TIMP-2 during retinal development but MMP-9 and TIMP-1 immunoreactivity of IPM of *wt* retina declined during development and Mueller cells completely lacked such staining at all time points. Such results suggest that MMP-2 and TIMP-2 might play a role in the maintenance of retinal integrity [65] in *wt* retina. The observation of MMP-2 and MMP-9 in OPL and in inner segments of IPM suggested that integrator neurons in PN14, -21 and -28 *wt* retinas expressed these MMPs for modification of IPM, whereas in the *rd1* retina intense expression of MMP-9 in OPL by integrator neurons could mean that MMP-9 contributes to its degeneration. RGC, Mueller cells and astrocytes show MMP-2, whereas GCL, IPM and retinal vasculature show mild MMP-9 reactivity in rat retina [22, 29]. On comparison with the meager information available from the literature, a species variation appears to exist in the cellular sources of MMP-2, MMP-9, cathepsin B, TIMP-1, TIMP-2 and cystatin C in the retina.

Higher Sialylation of Sgag In PN2, PN7 WT and PN7, PN14 Rd1 Retinas Respectively Indicated Neurogenesis in WT and Apoptosis In Rd1

The increased activity of the proteinases decreased the core protein part and increased the sGAG part of proteoglycans in *rd1* retina. This was also demonstrated by lectin blotting [6, 7 and 9], and is likely to give rise to an accumulation of low molecular weight sGAG in the ECM [6]. The weak staining for core proteins associated with the sGAG in proteoglycans band in the ECM and IPM of *rd1* retinal extracts suggested degradation of the core proteins which may predispose the photoreceptors to apoptosis [62]. The results of the present study show modification of proteoglycan saccharides in *rd1* retina and it has been reported that there is an association between defective glycosylation of proteoglycans and accumulation of secondary lysosomes and degeneration vacuoles along with alteration in collagen structure in the skin fibroblasts [97]. Higher sialylation of PN2 and PN7 *wt* but not of *rd1* along with higher galactosylation of proteoglycans at PN14 *rd1* could mean that the *rd1* retinal neurons were more susceptible to phagocytosis and apoptosis as reported for erythrocytes [10, 32 and 99] and neurons [67]; and *wt* retinal neurons were more responsive to neurogenesis and their axons to correct guidance cues for synaptogenesis at a specific age of development [17, 43, 67, 78, 108 and 118]. Delaying of such guidance cues in *rd1* retina may lead to a faulty and modified synaptogenesis between photoreceptors and RGC through the integrator neurons. This conclusion is supported by the observation of higher content of terminally desialylated and with exposed penultimate galactose of sGAG part of proteoglycans of erythrocyte and neurons, which are more prone to phagocytosis and apoptosis [10, 32, 67 and 99]. This may be related to the observations that terminal sialic acid residues mask the cells from recognition for phagocytosis by macrophages in blood, liver, spleen and CNS, whereas penultimate galactose exposed due to a lack of sialylation or after desialylation permits their recognition for phagocytosis and apoptosis. This view is supported by the report that the absence of polysialic acid increases apoptosis and decreases the survival of newly generated neurons in pre- and postnatal brain [67], whereas its presence promotes neurogenesis *in vitro* and *in vivo* [43, 108]. Thus desialylated *rd1* retinal neurons were probably more prone to apoptosis than to neurogenesis and the delayed development of neuronal processes generated faulty synaptogenesis between photoreceptors, integrator neurons and RGC in *rd1* retina.

Imbalance in Proteinases and their Inhibitors Lead to Degeneration in Rd1 Retina

MMPs have been implicated in remodeling of ECM for angiogenesis, signaling, arthritis, cancer and ECM degeneration during diseases of cardiovascular and central nervous systems [13, 119]. Whereas, TIMPs have been implicated in the inhibition of MMPs, cell signaling, growth and survival [13]. MMP-9 has been implicated activation of cell signaling and promotion of Schwann cell migration by binding of its hemopexin domain to low-density lipoprotein receptor-related protein. The signaling function of MMP-9 is independent of its proteinase activity. On its own the hemopexin domain of MMP-9 can participate in such signaling [130]. During the present studies it was observed that the *rd1* retina had decreased levels of proteins at PN21 and PN28 and proportionally higher levels and activities of sGAg, MMP-9, MMP-2, cathepsin B, -S and -L than those of concomitantly elevated proteinase inhibitors TIMP-1, TIMP-2 and cystatin C. These results suggested degradation of cellular and ECM proteins and further indicated that there was greater involvement of MMP-9 and cathepsin B in the degeneration of *rd1* retina. The role of serine proteinases in retinal physiopathology is still to be investigated to determine its place in proteinase hierarchy for their role in retinal degenerations.

Cathepsins possibly continue and complete the hydrolysis of ECM components initiated by MMPs. Cathepsin L, being 10-100 fold more active than cathepsin B on most substrates [16, 56] and being protected and activated by sGAG at neutral pH, it would bring about faster and intense degeneration of cell and ECM associated molecules in *rd1* retina at PN21 and PN28 stages of development. Unlike cathepsin L and cathepsin B, cathepsin S has narrow substrate specificity at neutral pH [16] and will further increase the rate and range of cleavage of cell and ECM components. These observations are in agreement with the role of MMPs and cathepsins in the degradation of ECM, inflammation and angiogenesis reported in other tissues [27]. MMP-9 upregulation increases the biosynthesis of heparin sulfate proteoglycans and a glycoprotein [61]. It also degrades laminin in the ECM; promotes death of RGC [53, 72] as well as retinal degeneration and loss of photoreceptors, irrespective of the cause and the species [121]. Both MMPs and cysteine cathepsins process a wide range of ECM-membrane-associated and cytosolic molecules including insulin, proteinases, bFGF, vascular endothelial growth factor (VEGF), actin, myosin, vimentin, collagens, proteoglycans, tubulin, glycoproteins and histones for physiopathological angiogenesis, tissue degeneration and neuronal cell death [16, 40, 56, 64 and 116]. MMPs are extracellular endopeptidases capable of catalyzing the partial hydrolysis of collagens to generate angiogenic endostatins which can be further degraded by endo- and exopeptidase cathepsin B but not by MMPs [40, 64 and 116]. Thus MMPs not only generate space for accommodating the developing blood vessels and neuronal processes but also provide angiogenic endostatins and play a hierarchical role during angiogenesis, healing and degeneration of the retina. In other tissues like mucosa and dermis also, the proteinases uPA, separase (a serine proteinase) and a number of MMPs (MMP-1, -9, -10, -12, -13, -14 and -3 and TIMP-1, -2, and -3) function in a collective and sequential and hierarchical manner for successful remodeling of ECM during wound healing [104]. By using short interference RNA (siRNA) it has been demonstrated that MMPs have autocrine action. MMP-9 increases apoptosis and decreases viability of keratinocytes through increased activity of phosphorylated p-38 protein, whereas MMP-2 does the opposite by increasing the activity of keratin-14 and phosphorylated extracellular signal-regulated kinase-2 (ERK2)[124]. Using inhibitors to prevent apoptosis in hepatocytes Dunstl et al. [131] reported that complete inhibition of apoptosis requires both cysteine proteinase inhibitor zVAD-fmk and serine proteinase inhibitors TLCK (N,p-tosyl-L-lysine chloromethyl ketone) and TPCK (N,α-tosyl-L-phenylalanine chloromethyl ketone).. This suggested that apoptosis like death of hepatocytes can take place due to cysteine proteinases caspases and in a caspase independent manner in presence of serine proteinase..

Proteinases Increased by TGF-B1 Activate it in Wt But Degrade it in Rd1 Retina

Due to a mutation in the β subunit of PDE the *rd1* retina has an inactive PDE which has been reported to result in an elevation of the levels of cGMP, ROS, Ca^{2+} ions, retinal blood vessels narrowing and deficiency as well as almost complete loss of rod photoreceptors [39, 58, 74 and 110]. The *rd1* retina shows oxidative stress which may be the consequence of hypoxia after narrowing and deficiency of blood vessels and lower levels of GPx and GST [8, 9] and this could be instrumental for the observed imbalances in the MMPs-TIMPs and cathepsins-cystatin C axes in favor of the proteinases. Activation of MMPs and cathepsins by superoxide has also been reported during myocardial remodeling [26, 83]. TGF-β_1 expressed by RPE, photoreceptors, Mueller glia cells, ganglion cells, astrocytes, hyalocytes and cells associated with choroidal and retinal blood vessels of mammalian retina transiently induces MMP-9 during retinal angiogenesis when ECM turnover is greatly accelerated [11, 15 and 60]. This is achieved by linking free TGF-β_1 to ECM through integrin $\alpha_3\beta_1$ [60]. Cytokines increase the expression of *Mmp* genes through the transcription factor c-Fos activation protein-1 (c-Fos/AP-1) [4].

TGF-β is known to have a Ca^{2+} stabilizing effect after Ca^{2+} overloading of the neurons [90] possibly by preservation of mitochondrial function [89] and by upregulating the expression of Na^+/Ca^{2+} exchanger protein [23]. Thus the increase in Ca^{2+} levels reported in *rd1* retina [39] may at least in part be explained by mitochondrial dysfunction and decreased levels of TGF-β_1 as a result of its lowered expression or increased degradation. Both endogenous and exogenous TGF-β_1 decrease the expression of iNOS in RPE cells which subsequently decreases the production of NO [107]. Low level of exogenous NO perturbs and suppresses the expression of endogenous TIMP-1 and may thus in turn increase the activity of MMP-9. TGF-β_1 also enhances expression of cathepsin B in myeloid tumor cell lines [33, 92], whereas TGF-β_2 expression and secretion is increased in cultured human optic nerve head astrocytes under conditions of oxidative stress [120]. Higher levels of TGF-β_1 in RCM secreted by PN7 *wt* explants may, therefore, be responsible for the transient increase in MMP-9 activities for ECM remodeling, for angiogenesis and neuronal restructuring in *wt* retina during early postnatal development. Same may be the case for higher and transient increase in cathepsin B in *wt* explants [7] due to enhanced expression of cathepsin B by TGF-β_1 as reported in myeloid tumor cell lines [33, 92]. The lower level of TGF-β_1 with higher activity of MMP-9 and cathepsin B in retinal extracts and in RCM [6, 7, 9 and the present study] secreted by *rd1* retina may be due to its degradation by increased levels of proteinases [84].

The higher ratio of active MMPs and cathepsins to their endogenous inhibitors TIMPs and cystatin C secreted by inner retina indicated that in spite of higher secretion of TIMPs and cystatin C, *rd1* explants degenerate due to higher activities of MMP-9 and cathepsin B. Lower levels of TGF-β_1 secreted by *rd1* explants suggested that either expression of MMP-9 and cathepsin B in *rd1* retina was not regulated by TGF-β_1 as has been reported for MMP-9 in glial cell lines [15] or these proteinases degraded TGF-β_1 and lowered its levels. Increased secretion of MMPs and cathepsin B independent of TGF-β_1 action may also be explained by increased cGMP level in retina which suppresses TIMP-1 expression and creates an imbalance between MMPs (MMP-9, -1, and -13) and TIMP-1 favoring activities of MMPs and other proteinases [39, 93]. An imbalance *in vitro* and *in vivo* in MMP-9 / TIMP-1 and cathepsin / cystatin C axes with increased MMP-9 and cathepsin B activities as observed in *rd1* retinal extracts [6, 7 and 9] and in RCM from *rd1* retinal explants during this study could be explained by such a pathway perhaps involving increased levels of cGMP reported in *rd1* retina [39]. Such increase in cysteine cathepsin B activity by TGF-β_1 has been reported in myeloid tumor cells [33, 92]. Higher activities of MMPs especially in Mueller cells and of cathepsin B in *rd1* retina [6, 7, 9 and present study] possibly due to increased level of TGF-β_1 lead to accumulation of sGAG [6] after degradation of protein part of proteoglycans of ECM. Accumulation of sGAG could hinder the healing processes and the movement of Mueller cells in degenerating retina [98]. Degradation of ECM by MMPs and cathepsins may also destroy the matrix-trophic coupling between endothelial cells and neurons and hinder the neuroprotection provided by BDNF secreted by endothelial cells via such matrix-trophic coupling [47]. BDNF is degraded by MMPs [31, 38] and degradation of BDNF, blood vessel deficiency and consequently decreased matrix-trophic coupling in *rd1* retina may thus predispose it to a deficiency of BDNF. This may explain the mechanism of effects of BDNF plus CNTF to rescue the rod photoreceptors reported in *rd1* retina [12].

Rescue of Photoreceptors by Rational Treatment of Rd1 Retina with Proteinases Inhibitors and Antioxidants

Treatment of retinitis pigmentosa with gene therapy would be a rational approach. However, such approaches are in an experimental stage and therefore, other rational approaches based on biochemical basis of pathogenesis of retinal degeneration also need to be investigated. Our studies bring out the importance of oxidative stress, cytokines and proteinases in the pathogenesis of retinitis pigmentosa. Therefore, the studies on the use of antioxidants and inhibitors of proteinases and cytokines in the treatment of retinal degeneration(s) may thus be in the right direction for the rescue of photoreceptors under degenerative and oxidative stress.

Proteinase inhibitors to rescue Rd1 rod photoreceptor

Generation of cytokines and proteinases like MMPs is important in the pathogenesis of inflammatory and degenerative diseases and is under the direct control of transcription factor c-Fos/AP-1. As compared to cancer of different tissues, vascular and inflammatory diseases are better candidates for treatment with orally administered inhibitors of MMPs because the latter diseases show genetic stability [60]. Inhibition of constitutive and individual proteinases may not be an effective approach because of the compensatory effect of other proteinases [45, 51 and 68]. T5224 or other broad spectrum inhibitors of c-Fos/AP-1 found successful during the experimental arthritis in mice by decreasing the level of MMPs and cytokines [4, 38, 51 and 63] need to be evaluated in the rescue of rods lost during retinal degenerations. Our studies demonstrate the involvement of TGF-β_1, MMPs and cathepsins in the development of retinal degeneration and suggest that inhibition of proteinases for the treatment of retinal degenerations is worth further investigation.

GST or a combination of antioxidants rescued Rd1 rod photoreceptor

Throughout its life, the retina generates free radicals by extensive exposure to light and oxygen and it does so at a higher level during disease situations. The oxidative stress thus produced degenerates the photoreceptors [18, 37, 48, 54, 55 and 112] which could be rescued partially by *in vivo* and *in vitro* administration of an antioxidant enzyme GST or a combination of antioxidants namely lutein, zeaxanthin, GSH and α-lipoic acid orally to *rd1* mice and added to the medium used to culture *rd1* retinal explants *in vitro* [8,

96]. The water solubility of GSH and oil solubility of other antioxidants had the advantage that these could be administered orally and without the need to use organic solvents for solublization or administration by injection as reported by other workers [57, 58]. The rescue effect was evident both with respect to a higher number of rows of surviving photoreceptors and a lower number of cells displaying DNA oxidatively damaged by free radicals during oxidative stress in *rd1* retinas. The rescue effect was better in PN17 than in PN11 *rd1* mouse retinas exposed to antioxidants from the PN3 stage. Although each of the antioxidants used during the study is potent scavenger of ROS yet individually these were ineffective in rescuing the photoreceptors. It is possible that the presence of water soluble GSH maintained the other antioxidants in reduced state after administration and improved their efficacy individually or collectively as antioxidants. Increased free radicals (ROS and RNS) activate MMPs and poly (ADP-ribose) polymerase (PARP) and inactivate a number of mitochondrial enzymes [26, 83]. PARP increases expression of inflammation causing genes and decreases NAD^+ and ATP along with release of free poly (ADP-ribose) polymers which affect mitochondrial function [83]. It is in this context interesting to note that the degenerating photoreceptors of the *rd1* retina have been shown to display increased PARP activity [87]. Low availability of GSH after oxidative injury activates caspase-9 and caspase-3 followed by PARP cleavage [20], although the cell death by caspases is not considered the sole pathway for *rd1* degeneration and is debatable [87]. The administration of these antioxidants to *rd1* mice may thus protect retinal cell DNA, RNA, plasma membranes and membranes of cell organelles namely mitochondria, lysosomes, GA and ER from oxidative damage and decrease the release of cathepsins, Ca^{2+} ions and free radicals. Decrease in Ca^{2+} ions lowers the calpain activity [77] and may control the vicious cycle for the release of cathepsins.

From the review of literature and from our own studies [6, 7, 8, 9, 96 and present study] it appears that after the failure of the primary antioxidant defense response, the secondary defense responses namely heat shock proteins, antioxidant enzymes and proteinases provide protection against free radicals by reversing the effects of oxidation and by degrading the oxidized proteins. Failure of such a response is followed by an increase in the levels of prosurvival factors to counteract the oxidative stress. If the stress still persists, the imbalance in the activities of proteinases and their endogenous inhibitors leads to degeneration and the disease condition.

Conclusion

The delayed sialylation or early desialylation of sGAG proteoglycans from PN2 and PN7 to PN14 stage of development in the *rd1* retina suggested that *rd1* neuronal cells were more susceptible to PCD, phagocytosis and apoptosis and to the generation of faulty and delayed axon guidance cues for differential synaptogenesis between the photoreceptors, integrating neurons and RGC. The transient imbalance in proteinases namely MMP-9 and cathepsin B and their endogenous inhibitors TIMP-1 and cystatin C in favor of proteinases in *wt* retina possibly remodels ECM and IPM for development of vascular and neuronal processes, whereas persistence of such an imbalance contributed by inner retina including Mueller cells in *rd1* retina produced degenerative changes. The transiently increased activities of MMPs and cathepsin B in RCM from *wt* explants were regulated by increase in the levels of TGF-β_1 and suggested proteolytic activation of TGF-β_1 [19, 109] and remodeling of ECM [6]. Whereas, persistently increased activities of MMPs and cathepsins, in spite of higher secretion of TIMPs and cystatin C into RCM by *rd1* explants were either not regulated by TGF-β_1 or TGF-β_1 expression was increased along with its degradation and that of ECM which also could contribute to the cell death [6, 7 and 84]. It was concluded that the PDE mutation in *rd1* mouse, leads to elevated levels of cGMP and ROS concentration which increased the free Ca^{2+} ions, calpain activity, lysosomal cathepsins and MMPs. This vicious cycle of an increase in calpain, cathepsins and MMPs activities, damages the organization of ECM, plasma membranes and cell organelles and releases of cathepsins, Ca^{2+} ions and ROS in *rd1* retinas. Importantly the rod photoreceptors in *rd1* retina were rescued to a limited extent, both by *in vitro* and *in vivo* treatments with a combination of antioxidants namely lutein, xeaxanthin, GSH and α-lipoic acid but GST alone also rescued the photoreceptors. Individually these antioxidants did not show protective effect for rod photoreceptors. Thus there is still a scope for improving the rescue of rod photoreceptors by treatment(s) with low molecular weight synthetic broad spectrum proteinase inhibitors on their own and / or in combination with antioxidants.

Future line of work involves delineating the status of oxidative stress in the retinal mitochondria and the distribution of proteinases (namely cathepsins, calpains, MMPs and serine proteinases) and their respective endogenous inhibitors (namely cystatin C, calpastatin, TIMPs and serpins) in retinas of living animals. This will give an idea of the real life status of these molecules. Such studies will be carried out by intravenous injections of synthetic, low molecular weight, membrane permeable fluorescent labeled probes (proteinase substrates and inhibitors, mitochondrial membrane potential detecting probes) and by tracing the retained fluorescence by whole animal imaging as well as by monitoring the fluorescence in retinas in frozen sections, in cell suspensions of mildly homogenized retinas. Similar approaches have been used to assess neuronal cell death in live animal brains [132]

Acknowledgments

Thanks are due to Inger Holmqvist (presently at the Department of Zoology, Göteborg University, Göteborg, Sweden); Anne-Catherine Löfström, Division of Clinical Chemistry and Pharmacology, Lund University Hospital; Birgitta Klefbohm, Hodan Abdalle and Katarina Said, Ophthalmology Department of Clinical Sciences, Lund University, for technical assistance and animal care; to Mattias Belting, Oncology Department, Lund University, for the use of the microplate fluorometer facility; to Dutch Retina Foundation (The Netherlands) and Foundation Fighting Blindness (U.S.A.) for financial support; and to the publishers of Ophthalmic Research (S. Karger, Medical and Scientific Publishers, Basel, Switzerland) and Investigative Ophthalmology and Visual Science (IOVS Editorial Office, Rockville, USA) for the permission to use data from figures published in our articles given as references 6 and 7, respectively. The Figures 4, 5, 7, 9 and Figures 6, 10 were modified from the pictures / data presented in Figures of references 6 and 7, respectively.

Disclosure

The authors indicate no potential conflicts of interest.

References

[1]   Abrahamson, M., Buttle, D. J., Mason, R. W., Hansson, H., Grubb, A., Lilja, H. & Ohlsson, K. M. (1991). Regulation of cystatin C activity by serine proteinases. *Biomed. Biochem Acta.*, *50*, 587-593.

[2]   Acosta, M. L., Fletcher, E. L., Azizoglu, S., Foster, L.E., Farber, D. B. & Kalloniatis, M. (2005). Early markers of retinal degeneration in rd/rd mice. *Mol. Vis. 11*, 717-728.

[3]   Agapova, O. A., Ricard, C. S., Salvador-Silva, M. & Harnendez, M. R. (2001). Expression of matrix metalloproteinases and tissue inhibitors of metalloproteinases in human optic nerve head astrocytes. *Glia.*, *33*, 205-216.

[4]   Aikawa, Y., Morimoto, K., Yamamoto, T., Chaki, H., Hashiramoto, A., Narita, H., Hirono, S. & Shiozawa, S. (2008). Treatment of arthritis with a selective inhibitor of c-Fos/activator protein-1. *Nature Biotech.*, *26*, 817-823.

[5]   Aiping, Z., Shuiqing, Z., Yang, C. & Qing, X. (2006). Modulation of matrix metalloproteinase and TIMP-1 expression by TGF-β_1 in cultured human RPE cells. *J. Huazhong Uni. Sci. Technol. [Med. Sci.]*, *26*, 363-365.

[6]   Ahuja, S., Ahuja, P., Caffe, A. R., Ekstrom, P., Abrahamson, M. & van Veen, T. (2006). rd1 mouse retina shows imbalance in cellular distribution and levels of TIMP-1/MMP-9, TIMP-2/MMP-2 and sulfated glycosaminoglycans. *Ophthalmic Res.*, *38*, 125-136.

[7]   Ahuja, S., Ahuja-Jensen, P., Johnson, L. E., Caffe, A. R., Abrahamson, M., Ekstrom, P. A. R. & van Veen, T. (2008). rd1 mouse retina shows an imbalance in the activity of cysteine protease cathepsins and their endogenous inhibitor cystatin C. *Invest. Ophthalmol. Vis. Res.*, *49*, 1089-1096.

[8]   Ahuja, P., Caffe, A. R., Ahuja, S., Ekström, P. & Van Veen, T. (2005). Decreased glutathione transferase levels in rd1/rd1 mouse retina: replenishment protects photoreceptors in retinal explants. *Neurosci.*, *131*, 935-943.

[9]   Ahuja-Jensen, P., Johnsen-Soriano, S; Ahuja, S., Bosch-Morell, F., Sancho-Tello, M., Romero, F. J., Abrahamson, M. & van Veen, T. (2007). Low glutathione peroxidase in rd1 mouse retina increases oxidative stress and proteases. *NeuroReport.*, *18*, 797-801.

[10] Aminoff, D., Bruegge, W. F. V., Bell, W. C., Sarpolis, K. & Williams, R. (1977). Role of sialic acid in survival of erythrocytes in the circulation: interaction of neuramindase-treated and untreated erythrocytes with spleen and liver at the cellular level. *Proc. Natl. Acad. Sci.*, U.S.A., *74*, 1521-1524.

[11] Anderson, D. H., Guerin, C. J., Hageman, G. S., Pfeffer, B. A. & Flanders, K. C. (1995). Distribution of transforming growth factor-beta isoforms in the mammalian retina. *J. Neurosci. Res.*, *42*, 63-79.

[12] Azadi, S., Johnson, L. E., Paquet-Durand, F., Perez, M. T., Zhang, Y., Ekström, P. A. R. & van Veen, T. (2007). CNTF-BDNF treatment and neuroprotective pathways in rd1 mouse retina, *Brain Res.*, *1129*, 116-129.

[13] Baker, A. H., Edwards, D. R. & Murphy, G. (2002). Metalloproteinase inhibitors: biological actions and therapeutic opportunities. *J. Cell Sci.*, *115*, 3719-3727.

[14] Beier, M., Franke, A., Paunel-Gorgulu, A. N., Scheere, N. & Dunker, N. (2006) Transforming growth factor beta mediates apoptosis in the ganglion cell layer during all programmed cell death periods of developing murine retina. *Neurosci. Res.*, *56*, 193-203.

[15] Behzadian, M. A., Wang, X. L., Windsor, L. J., Ghaly, N. & Caldwell, R. B. (2001). TGF β increases retinal endothelial cell permeability by increasing MMP-9: possible role of glial cells in endothelial barrier function. *Invest. Ophthalmol. Vis. Sci.*, *42*, 853-859.

[16] Bohley, P. & Seglen, P. O. (1992). Proteases and proteolysis in the lysosome. *Experientia.*, *48*, 151-157.

[17] Bonfanti, L. (2006). PSA-NCAM in mammalian structural plasticity and neurogenesis. *Prog. Neurobiol.*, *80*, 129-164.

[18] Bonne, C., Muller, A. & Villain, M. (1998). Free radicals in retinal ischemia. *Gen. Pharmac.*, *30*, 275-280.

[19] Bouvet, C., Moreau, S., Blanchette, J., de Blois, D. & Moreau, P. (2008). Sequential activation of matrix metalloproteinase 9 and transforming growth factor β in arterial elastocalcinosis. *Arterioscler. Thromb. Vasc. Biol.*, *28*, 856-862.

[20] Butts, B. D., Houde, C. & Mehmet, H. (2008). Maturation dependent sensitivity of oligodendrocyte lineage cells to apoptosis: implications for normal development and disease. *Cell Death Diff.*, *15*, 1178-1186.

[21] Caffe, A. R., Ahuja, P., Holmqvist, B., Azadi, S., Forsell, J., Holmqvist, I., Söderpalm, A. K. & van Veen, T. (2001). Mouse retina explants after

long-term culture in serum free medium. *J. Chem. Neuroanat.*, *22*, 263-273.

[22] Canete-Soler, R., Gui, Y. H., Linask, K. K. & Muschel, R. J. (1995). MMP-9 (gelatinase B) mRNA is expressed during mouse neurogenesis, and may be associated with vascularization. *Brain Res. Dev. Brain Res.*, *88*, 37-52.

[23] Carrillo, C., Cafferata, E. G., Genovese, J., O´Reilly, M., Roberts, A. B. & Santa-Coloma, T. A. (1998). TGF β_1 up-regulates the mRNA for the Na+/Ca2+ exchanger in neonatal rat cardiac myocytes. *Cell Mol. Biol.*, *44*, 543-551.

[24] Chakraborti, S. Mandal, M. Das, S. Mandal, A. & Chakraborti, T. (2003). Regulation of matrix metalloproteinases: an overview. *Mol. Cell. Biochem.*, *253*, 269-285.

[25] Chang, B. Hawes, N. L. Hurd, R. E. Davisson, M. T. Nusinowitz, S. & Heckenlively, J. R. (2002) Retinal degeneration mutants in the mouse. *Vis. Res.*, *42*, 517-525.

[26] Cheng, X. W., Murohara, T., Kuzuya, M., Izawa, H., Sasaki. T., Obata, K., Nagata, K., Nishizawa, T., Kobayashi, M., Yamada, T., Kim, W., Sato, K., Shi, G. P., Okumura, K. & Yokota M. (2008). Superoxide-dependent cathepsin activation is associated with hypertensive myocardial remodeling and represents a target for angiotensin II type 1 receptor blocker treatment. *Am. J. Pathol.*, *173*, 358-369.

[27] Chapman, H. A., Riese, R. J. & Shi, G. P. (1997). Emerging roles of cysteine proteases in human biology. *Ann. Rev. Physiol.*, *59*, 63-88.

[28] Chintala, S. K. (2006). The emerging role of proteases in retinal ganglion cell death. *Exp. Eye Res.*, *82*, 5-12.

[29] Chintala, S. K., Zhang, X., Austin, J. S. & Fini, M. E. (2002). Deficiency in matrix metalloproteinase gelatinase B (MMP-9) protects against retinal ganglion cell death after optic nerve ligation. *J. Biol. Chem.*, *277*, 47461-47468.

[30] Chwieralski, C. E., Welte, T. & Bühling, F. (2006). Cathepsin-regulated apoptosis. *Apoptosis.*, *11*, 143-149.

[31] Cuzner, M. L. & Opdenakker, G. (1999). Plasminogen activators and matrix metalloproteases, mediators of extracellular proteolysis in inflammatory demyelination of the central nervous system. *J Neuroimmunol.*, *94*, 1-14.

[32] Durocher, J. R., Payne R. C. & Conrad, M. E. (1975). Role of sialic acid in erythrocyte survival. *Blood.*, *45*, 11-20.

[33]   Dawley, W. P., Peters, S. B. & Larsen, M. (2008). Extracellular matrix dynamics in development and regenerative medicine. *J. Cell Sci.*, *121*, 255-264.

[34]   Decanini, A., Nordgaard, C. L., Feng, X. Ferrington, D. A. & Olsen, T. W. (2007). Changes in select redox proteins, of the retinal pigment epithelium in age related macular degeneration. *Am. J. Ophthalmol.*, *143*, 607-615.

[35]   De Vos, K. J., Grierson, A. J., Ackerley, S. & Miller, C. C. (2008). Role of axonal transport in neurodegenerative diseases. *Annu Rev Neurosci.*, *31*, 151-173.

[36]   Dong, A., Shen, J., Krause, M., Akiyama, H., Hackett, S. F., Lai, H. & Campochiaro, P. A. (2006). Superoxide dismutase 1 protects retinal cells from oxidative damage. *J. Cell. Physiol.*, *208*, 516-526.

[37]   Dringen, R. (2005). Oxidative and anti-oxidative potential of brain microglial cells. *Antioxidants Redox Signaling.*, *7*, 1223-2331.

[38]   Ethell, I. M. & Ethell, D. W. (2007). Matrix metalloproteinases in brain development and remodeling: synaptic functions and targets. *J. Neurosci. Res.*, *85*, 2813-2823.

[39]   Farber, D. B., Flannery, J. G., and Bowesrickman C. (1994). The rd mouse story: Seventy years of research on an animal model of inherited retinal degeneration. *Prog. Retinal Eye Res.*, *13*, 31-64.

[40]   Ferreras, M., Felbor, U., Lenhard, T., Olsen, B. R. & Delaisse, J. (2000). Generation and degradation of human endostatin proteins by various proteinases. *FEBS Lett.*, *486*, 247-251.

[41]   Ganea, E. & Harding, J. J. (2006). Glutathione related enzymes and the eye. *Curr. Eye Res.*, *31*, 1-11.

[42]   Gao, F., Koenitzer, J. R., Tobolewski, J. M., Jiang, D., Liang, J., Noble, P. W. & Oury, T. D. (2008). Extracellular Superoxide dismutase inhibits inflammation by preventing oxidative fragmentation of hyaluronan. *J. Biol. Chem.*, *283*, 6058-6066.

[43]   Gascon, E., Vutskits, L. & Kiss, J. Z. (2008). The role of PSA-NCAM in adult neurogenesis. *Neurochem. Res. May 31.*, (Epub ahead of print).

[44]   Geraghty, P., Rogan, H. P., Greene, C. M., Boxio, R. M., Poiriert, T., O'Mahony, M., Belaaouaj, A., O'Neill. S. J., Taggart, C. C. & McElvaney, N. G. (2007). Neutrophil elastase up-regulates cathepsin B and matrix metalloprotease-2 expression. *J. Immunol.*, *178*, 5871-5878.

[45]   Green, K. A., Almholt, K., Ploug, M., Rønø, B., Castellino, F. J., Johnsen, M., Bugge, T. H. & Rømer J., Lund L. R. (2008).

Profibrinolytic effects of metalloproteinases during skin wound healing in the absence of plasminogen. *J Invest Dermatol.*, *128*, 2092-2101.

[46] Guerin, C. J., Hu, L., Scicli, G. & Scicli, G. (2001). Transforming growth factor beta in experimentally detached retina and periretinal membranes. *Exp. Eye Res. 73.*, 753-764.

[47] Guo, S., Kim, W. J., Lok, J., Lee, S. R., Besancon, E., Luo, B. H., Stins, M. F., Wang, S., Dedhar, S. & Lo, E. H. (2008). Neuroprotection via matrix-trophic coupling between cerebral endothelial cells and neurons. *Proc. Natl. Acad. Sci. U.S.A.*, *105*, 7582-7587.

[48] Halliwell B. & Gutteridge, J. M. C. Free radicals in biology and medicine. Oxford U.K.: Oxford University Press; 2007.

[49] Hasegawa, A., Naruse, M., Hitoshi, S., Iwasaki, S., Takebayashi, H. & Ikenaka, K. (2007). Regulation of glial development by cystatin C. *J. Neurochem.*, *100*, 12-22.

[50] Honjo, Y., Nagineni, C. N., Larsson, J., Nandula, S. R., Hooks, J. J., Chan, C. C., Karlsson, S. & Kulkarni, A. B. (2007). Neuron-specific TGF-β signaling deficiency results in retinal detachment and cataracts in mice. *Biochem. Biophys. Res. Commun.*, *352* 418-422.

[51] Hu, J., van den Steen, P. E., Sang, Q. X. A. & Opdenakker, G. (2007). Matrix metalloproteinase inhibitors as therapy for inflammatory and vascular diseases. *Nature Rev. Drug Discovery.*, *6*, 480-498.

[52] Jain, A., Fisher, L. W. & Fedarko, N. S. (2008). Bone sialoprotein binding to matrix metalloproteinase-2 alters enzyme inhibition kinetics. *Biochemistry.*, *47*, 5986-5995.

[53] Jones, B. W., Watt, C. B., Frederick, J. M., Baehr, W., Chen, C. K., Levine, E. M., Milam, A. H., LeVail, M. M. & Marc, R. E. (2003). Retinal remodeling triggered by photoreceptor degeneration. *J. Comp. Neurol.*, *464*, 1-16.

[54] Jones, D. P. (2006). Redefining oxidative stress, Antioxidants. *Redox Signaling.*, *8*, 1865-1879.

[55] Jones, D. P. (2006). Extra-cellular redox state: refining the definition of oxidative stress in aging. *Rejuvenation Res.*, *9*, 169-181.

[56] Kirschke, H., Barrett, A. J. & Rawlings, N. D. (1995). Proteinases 1: lysosomal cysteine proteinases. *Protein Profile.*, *2*, 1581-1643.

[57] Komeima, K., Rogers, B. S. & Campochiaro, P. A. (2007). Antioxidants slow photoreceptor cell death in mouse models of retinitis pigmentosa. *J. Cell. Physiol.*, *213*, 809-815.

[58] Komeima, K., Rogers, B. S., Lu, L. & Campochiaro, P. A. (2006). Antioxidants reduce cone cell death in a model of retinitis pigmentosa. *Proc. Natl. Acad. Sci. U.S.A.*, *103*, 11300-11305.

[59] Laemmli, U. K. (1970). Cleavage of structural proteins during the assembly of the head of bacteriophage T4. *Nature.*, *227*, 680-685.

[60] Lamar, J. M., Iyer, V. & DiPersio, C. M. (2008). Integrin $\alpha_3\beta_1$ potentiates TGF β-mediated induction of MMP-9 in immortalized keratinocytes. *J. Invest. Dermatol.*, *128*, 575-586.

[61] Landers, R. A., Rayborn, M. E. & Myers, K. M. (1994). Increased retinal synthesis of heparin sulfate proteoglycan and HNK-1 glycoproteins following photoreceptor degeneration. *J. Neurochem.*, *93*, 737-750.

[62] Lazarus, H. S., Sly, W. S., Kyle, J. W. & Hageman, G. S. (1993). Photoreceptor degeneration and altered distribution of interphotoreceptor matrix proteoglycans in the mucopolysaccharidosis VII mouse. *Exp. Eye Res.*, *56*, 531-541.

[63] Levicar, N., Nutali, R. K. & Lah, T. T. (2003). Proteases in brain tumour progression, *Acta Neurochir.*, *145*, 825-838..

[64] Li, Z., Yasuda, Y., Li, W., Bogyo, M., Katz, N., and Gordon, R. E., Fields, G. B. & Brömme, D. (2004). Regulation of collagenase activities of human cathepsins by glycosaminoglycans. *J. Biol. Chem.*, *279*, 5470-5479.

[65] Limb, G. A., Daniels, J. T., Pleass, R., Charteris, D. G., Luthert, P. J. & Khaw, P. T. (2002). Differential expression of matrix metalloproteinases 2 and 9 by glial Mueller cells response to soluble and extracellular matrix-bound tumor factor-alpha. *Am. J. Pathol.*, *160*, 1847-1855.

[66] Liu, N., Raja, S. M., Zazzeroni, F., Metkar, S. S., Shah, R., Zhang, M., Wang, Y., Brömme, D., Russin, W. A., Lee, J. C., Peter, M. E., Froelich, C. J., Franzoso, G. & Ashton-Rickardt P.G. (2003). NF-kappaB protects from the lysosomal pathway of cell death. *EMBO J.*, *22*,:5313-22.

[67] Lossi, L. & Merighi, A. (2003). In vivo cellular and molecular mechanisms of neuronal apoptosis in the mammalian CNS. *Prog. Neurobiol.*, *69*, 287-312.

[68] Lund, L. R., Romer, J., Bugge, T. H., Nielsen., Frandsen, T. L., Degen, J. L., Stephens, R. W. & Danø, K. (1999). Functional overlap between two classes of matrix-degrading proteases in wound healing. *EMBO J.*, *18*,:4645-4656.

[69] Maier, P., Broszinski, A., Heizmann, U. & Reinhard, T. (2008). Decreased active TGF-β_2 levels in the aqueous humour during immune reactions following penetrating keratoplasty. *Eye 22*, 569-575.

[70] Mali, R. S., Cheng, M. & Chintala, S. K. (2005) Plasminogen activators promote excitotoxicity-induced retinal damage. *FASEB J.*, *19*, 1280-1289.

[71] Mandelker, L. (2008). Introduction to oxidative stress and mitochondrial dysfunction. *Vet. Clinics North Am.: Small Anim. Practice 38*, 1-30.

[72] Marc, R. E., Jones, B. W., Watt, C. B. & Strettoi, E. (2003). Neural remodeling in retinal degeneration. *Prog. Retina Eye Res.*, *22*, 607-655.

[73] Masson, V. (2006). Roles of serine proteases and matrix metalloproteinases in tumor invasion and angiogenesis. *Bull. Mem. Acad. R. Med. Belg.*, *161*, 320-326.

[74] Matthes, M. T. & Bok, D (1984). Blood vascular abnormalities in the degenerative mouse retina (C57BL/6J-rd Ie). *Invest. Ophthalmol. Vis. Sci.*, *25*, 364-369.

[75] McLaughlin, M. E., Ehrhart, T. L.,Berson, E. L. & Dryja, T. P. (1995). Mutation spectrum of the gene encoding the beta subunit of rod phosphodiesterase among patients with autosomal recessive retinitis pigmentosa. *Proc. Natl. Acad. Sci. U.S.A.*, *92*, 3249-3253.

[76] Meran, S., Thomas, D. W., Stephens, P., Enoch, S., Martin, J., Steadman, R. & Phillips, A.O (2008). Hyaluronan facilitates transforming growth factor-β_1-mediated fibroblast proliferation. *J. Biol. Chem. 283*, 6530-6545.

[77] Molinari, M., Anagli, J. & Carafoli, E. (1994). Ca^{2+}activated neutral protease is active in the erythrocyte membrane in its nonautolyzed 80-kDa form. *J Biol Chem.*, *269*, 27992-27995.

[78] Muller, D., Djebbara-Hannas, Z., Jourdain, P., Vutskits, L., Durbec, P., Rougon, G. & Kiss J.Z., (2000). Brain-derived neurotrophic factor restores long-term potentiation in polysialic acid-neural cell adhesion molecule-deficient hippocampus. *Proc. Natl. Acad. Sci. U.S.A.*, *97*, 4315-4320.

[79] Müller, E. , Schröder, C., Schauer, R. & Sharon, N. (1983).. Binding and phagocytosis of sialidase-treated rat erythrocytes by a mechanism independent of opsonins. *Hoppe Seylers Z. Physiol. Chem.*, 364, 1419-1429.

[80] Nakanishi, H. (2002). Microglial functions and proteases. *Mol. Neurobiol.*, *27*, 163-176.

[81] Nishiyama, K., Konishi, A., Nishio, C., Araki-Yoshida, K., Hatanaka, H., Kojima, M., Ohmiya Y., Yamada, M. & Koshimizu H. (2005). Expression of cystatin C prevents oxidative stress-induced death in PC12 cells. *Brain Res. Bull.*, *67*, 94-99.

[82] Packer, L. (1998). Alpha lipoic acid: a metabolic antioxidant which regulates NF-kappa B signal transduction and protects against oxidative injury. *Drug Metab. Rev.*, *30*, 245-275.

[83] Pacher, P. & Szabo, C. (2008). Role of peroxynitrite-poly (ADP-ribose) polymerase pathway in human disease. *Am. J. Pathol.*, *173*, 2-13.

[84] Paczek, L., Gaciong, Z., Bartlomiejczyk, I., Sebekova, K. & Birkenmeier, G. (2001). Protease administration decreases enhanced transforming growth factor-beta 1 content in isolated glomeruli of diabetic rats. *Drugs Exp. Clin. Res.*, *27*,141-149.

[85] Padgett, L. C., Lui, G. M., Werb, Z. & La Vail, M. M. (1997). Matrix metalloproteinase-2 and tissue inhibitor of metalloproteinase-1 in retinal pigment epithelium and interphotoreceptor matrix: vectorial secretion and regulation. *Exp. Eye Res. 64*, 927-938.

[86] Paquet-Durand, F., Azadi, S., Hauk, S.M., Ueffing, M., van Veen, T. & Ekström, P. (2006). Calpain is activated in degenerating photoreceptors in the rd1 mouse, *J. Neurochem.*, *96*, 802-814.

[87] Paquet-Durand, F., Silva, J., Talukdar, T., Johnson, L. E., Azadi, S., van Veen, T., Ueffing, M., Hauck, S.M. & Ekström PA. (2007). Excessive activation of poly(ADP-ribose) polymerase contributes to inherited photoreceptor degeneration in the retinal degeneration 1 mouse. *J. Neurosci.*, *27*, 10311-10319.

[88] Pilz, R. B. & Broderick, K. E. (2005). Role of cyclic GMP, in gene regulation. *Front. Biosci.*, *10*, 1239-1268.

[89] Prehn, J. H., Bindokas, V. P., Jordan, J., Galindo, M. F., Ghadge, G. D., Roos, R. P., Biose, L. H., Thompson, C. B., Krajewski, S., Reed, J. C. & Miller, R. J. (1996). Protective effect of transforming growth factor-beta 1 on beta-amyloid neurotoxicity in rat hippocampal neurons. *Mol. Pharmacol.*, *49*, 319-328.

[90] Prehn, J. H. M. & Miller, R. J. (1996). Opposite effects of TGF β_1 on rapidly- and slowly-triggered excitotoxic injury. *Neuropharmacol.*, *35*, 249-256.

[91] Pirttilä, T. J. Lukasiuk, K. Håkansson, K. Grubb, A. Abrahamson, M. & Pitkänen, A. (2005). Cystatin C modulates neurodegeneration and

neurogenesis following status epilepticus in mouse. *Neurobiol. Dis.*, *20*, 241-253.

[92] Reisenauer, A., Eickelberg, O., Wille, A., Heimburg, A., Reinhold, A., Sloane, B. F., Welte, T. & Buhling, F. (2007). Increased carcinogenic potential of myeloid tumor cells induced by aberrant TGF-β1 signaling and up regulation of cathepsin B. *Biol. Chem.*, *388*, 639-650.

[93] Ridnour, L. A., Windhausen, A. N., Isenberg, J. S., Yeung, N., Thomas, D. S., Vitek, M. P., Roberts, D. D. & Wink, D. A. (2007). Nitric oxide regulates matrix metalloproteinase-9 activity by guanyl-cyclase-dependent and –independent pathways. *Proc. Natl. Acad. Sci. U.S.A.*, *104*, 16898-16903.

[94] Roberts, A. B. (2003). Smoke signals for lung disease. *Nature 422*, 130-131.

[95] Sanyal, S. & Bal, A. K. (1973). Comparative light and electron microscopic study of retinal histogenesis in normal and rd mutant mouse. *Entwicklungsgesch.*, *142*, 219-238.

[96] Sanz, M. M. Johnson, L. E. Ahuja, S. Ekstrom, P. A. R. Romero, J. & van Veen, T. (2007). Significant photoreceptor rescue by treatment with a combination of antioxidants in an animal model for retinal degeneration. *Neurosci.*, *145*, 1120-1129.

[97] Seidler, D. G., Faiyaz-Ul-Haque, M., Hansen, U., Yip, G. W., Zaidi, S. H., Teebi, A. S., Kiesel, L. & Götte M. (2006). Defective glycosylation of decorin and biglycan, altered collagen structure, and abnormal phenotype of the skin fibroblasts of an Ehlers-Danlos syndrome patient carrying the novel Arg270Cys substitution in galactosyltransferase I (beta4GalT-7). *J. Mol. Med.*, *84*, 583-594.

[98] Singhal, S., Lawrence, J. M., Bhatia, B., Ellis, J. S., Kwan, A. S., MacNeil, A., Luthert, P. J., Fawcett, J. W., Perez, M. T., Khaw, P. T. & Limb. G. A. (2008). Chondroitin sulfate proteoglycans and microglia prevent migration and integration of grafted Mueller cells into degenerating ratina. *Stem Cells 26*, 1074-1082.

[99] Sinpitaksakul, S. N. Pimkhaokham, A. Sanchavanakit, N. & Pavasant, P. (2008). TGF-β1 induced MMP-9 expression in HNSCC cell lines via, Smad/MLCK pathway. *Biochem. Biophys. Res. Commun.*, *371*, 713-718.

[100] Sivak, J. M. & Fini, M. E. (2002). MMPs in the eye: emerging roles for matrix metalloproteinases in ocular physiology. *Prog. Retinal Eye Physiol.*, *21*, 1-14.

[101] Sokol, J. P. & Schiemann, W. P. (2004). Cystatin C antagonizes transforming growth factor beta signaling in normal and cancer cells. *Mol. Cancer Res.*, *2*, 183-195.

[102] Sommerburg, O. G., Siems, W. G., Hurst, J. S., Lewis, J. W., Kliger, D. S. & van Kuijk, F. J. (!999). Lutein and Zeaxanthin are associated with photoreceptors in human retina. *Curr. Eye Res.*, *19*, 491-495.

[103] Stahl W. & Sies, H. (2005). Bioactivity and protective effects of natural carotenoids. *Biochim. Biophys. Acta 1740*, 101-107. [100] Sivak, J.M. & Fini, M.E. (2002). MMPs in the eye: emerging roles for matrix metalloproteinases in ocular physiology. *Prog. Retinal Eye Physiol.*, *21*, 1-14.

[104] Steffensen, B. Hakkinen, L. & Larjava, H. (2001). Proteolytic events of wound healing- coordinated interactions among matrix metalloproteinases (MMPs), integrins, and extracellular matrix molecules. *Crit. Rev. Oral Biol. Med.*, *12*, 373-398.

[105] Sternlicht, M. D. & Werb, Z. (2001). How matrix metalloproteinases regulate cell behaviour. *Ann. Rev. Cell Dev. Biol.*, *17*, 463-513.

[106] Valentine, J. S. & Gralla, E. B. (2008). Introduction: reactive oxygen species special feature. *Proc. Natl. Acad. Sci. U.S.A.*, *105*, 8178-8178.

[107] Vodovotz, Y., Letterio, J. J., Geiser, A. G., Chesler, L., Roberts, A. B. & Sparrow, J. (1996). Control of nitric oxide production by endogenous TGF β_1 and systemic nitric oxide in retinal pigmented epithelial cells and peritoneal macrophages. *J. Leukoc. Biol.*, *60*, 261-270.

[108] Vutskits, L., Gascon, E., Zgraggen, E. & Kiss, J. Z. (2006). The polysialylated neural cell adhesion molecule promotes neurogenesis in vitro. *Neurochem. Res.*, *31*, 215-225.

[109] Wang, M. Zhao, D. Spinetti, G. Zhang, J. Jiang, L. Q. Pintus, G. Monticone, R. & Lakatta, E. G. (2006). Matrix metalloproteinase 2 activation of transforming growth factor- β_1 (TGF-β_1) and TGF-β_1-type II receptor signaling within the aged arterial wall. *Arterioscler. Thromb. Vasc. Biol.*, *26*, 1503-1509.

[110] Wang, S., Villegas-Perez, M. P., Vidal-Sanz, M. & Lund, R. D. (2000). Progressive optic axon dystrophy and vascular changes in *rd* mouse. *Invest. Ophthalmol. Vis. Sci.*, *41*, 537-545.

[111] Wang, X., Inoue, S., Gu, J., Miyoshi, E., Noda, K., Li, W., Mizuno-Horikawa, Y., Nakano, M., Takahashi, M., Uozumi, N., Ihara, S., Lee, S. H., Ikeda, Y., Yamaguchi, Y., Aze, Y., Tomiyama, Y., Fujii, J., Suzuki, K., Kondo, A., Shapiro, S. D., Lopez-Otin, C., Kuwaki, T.,

Okabe, M., Honke, K. & Taniguchi, N. (2005). Dysregulation TGF-β_1 receptor activation leads to abnormal lung development and emphysema-like phenotype in core fucose-deficient mice. *Proc. Natl. Acad. Sci. U.S.A.*, *102*, 15791-15796.

[112] Winterbourn, C. C. (2008). Reconsiling the chemistry and biology of reactive oxygen species. *Nature Chem. Biol.*, *4*, 278-286.

[113] Yamada, H., Obata, H., Kaji, Y. & Yamashita, H. (1999). Expression of transforming growth factor-β superfamily receptors in developing rat eyes. *Jpn. J. Ophthalmol.*, *43*, 290-294.

[114] Yafai, Y., Lange, J., Wiedemann, P., Reichenbach, A. & Eichler, W. (2007) Pigment epithelium derived factor acts as an opponent of growth stimulatory factors in retinal glial-endothelial cell interactions. *Glia 55*, 642-651.

[115] Yamamoto, N., Sawada, H., Izumi Y., Kume, T., Katsuki, H., Shimohama, S. & Akaike A. (2007). Proteasome inhibition induces glutathione synthesis and protects cells from oxidative stress: relevance to Parkinson Disease. *J. Biol. Chem.*, *282*, 4364-4372.

[116] Yamashima, T. (2000). Implication of cysteine proteases calpain, cathepsin and caspase in ischemic neuronal death of primates. *Prog. Neurobiol.*, *62*, 273-295.

[117] Yaun, L. & Neufeld, A. H. (2001). Activated microglia in the human glaucomatous optic nerve head. *J. Neurosci. Res.*, *64*, 523-532.

[118] Yin, X., Watanabe, M. & Rutishauser, U. (1995). Effect of polysialic acid on behavior of retinal ganglion cell axons during growth into the optic tract and tectum. *Development 121*, 3439-3446.

[119] Yong, V. W., Power, C., Forsyth, P. & Edwards, D. R. (2001). Metalloproteinases in biology and pathology of the nervous system. *Nature Rev Neurosci.*, *2*, 502-511.

[120] Yu, A. L., Fuchshofer, R., Birke, M., Kampik, A., Bloemendal, H. & Welge-Lussen, U. (2008). Oxidative stress and TGF-β2 increase heat shock protein 27 expression in human optic nerve head astrocytes. *Invest. Ophthalmol. Vis. Sci. Jun 14., [Epub ahead of print]*

[121] Zhang, X. Cheng, M. & Chintala, S. K. (2004). Kainic acid mediated up regulation of matrix metalloproteinase-9 promotes retinal degeneration. *Invest. Ophthalmol. Vis. Sci.*, *45*, 2374-2383.

[122] Quintanilla-Dieck, M. J., Codriansky, K., Keady, M., Bhawan, J. & Rünger, T. M. (2008). Cathepsin K in melanoma invasion. *J. Invest. Dermatol.,128, 2281-2288.*

[123] Han, Y. P., Yan, C. & Garner, W. L.. (2008) Proteolytic activation of matrix metalloproteinase-9 in skin wound healing is inhibited by alpha-1-antichymotrypsin.*J. Invest. Dermatol., 128, 2334-2342.*

[124] Xue, M, Jackson, C. J. (2008). Autocrine Actions of Matrix Metalloproteinase (MMP)-2 Counter the Effects of MMP-9 to Promote Survival and Prevent Terminal Differentiation of Cultured Human Keratinocytes. *J Invest Dermatol. May 22. [Epub ahead of print] PMID: 18496568 [PubMed - as supplied by publisher].*

[125] Bano, D, Munarriz, E., Chen, H. L., Ziviani, E., Lippi, G., Young, K. W. & Nicotera P. (2007). The plasma membrane Na+/Ca2+ exchanger is cleaved by distinct protease families in neuronal cell death. *Ann N Y Acad Sci., 1099, 451-455.*

[126] Bano, D., Young, K. W., Guerin, C. J., Lefeuvre, R., Rothwell, N. J., Naldini, L., Rizzuto, R., Carafoli, E., and Nicotera P. (2005). Cleavage of the plasma membrane Na+/Ca2+ exchanger in excitotoxicity. *Cell., 120, 275-285.*

[127] Schwab, B. L.., Guerini, D., Didszun, C., Bano, D., Ferrando-May, E., Fava E., Tam, J., Xu, D., Xanthoudakis, S., Nicholson, D. W., Carafoli, E. & Nicotera, P. (2002). Cleavage of plasma membrane calcium pumps by·caspases: a link between apoptosis and necrosis. *Cell Death Differ., 9, 818-831.*

[128] Pászty, K., Antalffy, G., Hegedüs, L., Padányi, R., Penheiter, A.R, Filoteo, A. G, Penniston, J. T. & Enyedi, A. (2007). Cleavage of the plasma membrane Ca+ATPase during apoptosis. *Ann N Y Acad Sci., 1099, 440-450.*

[129] Bano, D. & Nicotera, P. (2007). Ca2+ signals and neuronal death in brain ischemia.*Stroke., 38, 674-676.*

[130] Mantuano, E., Inoue, G., Li, X., Takahashi, K., Gaultier, A., Gonias S. L. & Campana, W. M. (2008). The hemopexin domain of matrix metalloproteinase-9 activates cell signaling and promotes migration of Schwann cells by binding to low-density lipoprotein receptor-related protein. *J. Neurosci., 28, 11571-11582.*

[131] Dünstl, G., Weiland, T., Schlaeger, C., Nüssler, A., Künstle, G. & Wendel, A.. (2007). Activation of an alternative death receptor-induced signaling pathway in human hepatocytes under caspase arrest. *Arch Biochem Biophys.,* Jun 15, *462, 140-149.*

[132] Anonymous. (2009). Fluorescent probes: neuroscience application guide., *Immunochemistry Technologies,* 1-16.

In: Reginitis Pigmentosa: Causes, Diagnosis...   ISBN: 978-1-60876-884-4
Editors: M. Baert, et al. pp. 191-208   © 2010 Nova Science Publishers, Inc.

Visual Training in Retinitis Pigmentosa Patients: Neural Plasticity and Function Recovery[*]

[1]Enzo M. Vingolo, [2]Serena Salvatore,
[3]Pier Luigi Grenga and [4]Paolo Limoli
[1]Department of Ophthalmology, University "La Sapienza" of Rome, Italy.
[2]Polo Pontino, Ospedale Alfredo Fiorini, Terracina, Italy.
[3]Centro Studi Ipovisione, Milan, Italy.
[4]Department of Ophthalmology, University "La Sapienza" of Rome, Italy.

Abstract

The aim of our study was to ascertain if visual training by means of Visual Pathfinder (LACE inc.) biofeedback system could be successful to improve and/or restore visual function in visually impaired patients with retinitis pigmentosa.

We enrolled 15 patients (age range 8-55) and examined a total of 30 eyes with retinitis pigmentosa. All the patients underwent a complete

---

[*] A version of this chapter was also published in Retinal Degeneration: Causes, Diagnosis and Treatment, edited by Robert B. Catlin, Nova Science Publishers. It was submitted for appropriate modifications in an effort to encourage wider dissemination of research.

ophthalmologic evaluation which comprised the assessment of best corrected visual acuity (BCVA) and pattern reversal visual evoked potential (VEP) according to the ISCEV standards. All the patients underwent 10 training sessions of 10 minutes each eye performed once a week using the Visual Pathfinder.

Statistical analysis was performed using the Student's t-test. P values less than 0.05 were considered statistically significant.

The mean BCVA was 0.67± 0.14 logMAR at the baseline assessment, and 0.84± 0.11 logMAR at the end of visual training; this result was statistically significant (p=0.035). VEP amplitude of P100 wave was 2.14±0.88 mV at the baseline assessment, and 4.86 ±1.12 mV at the end of visual training; this result was statistically significant (p=0.012).

In conclusion our experience demonstrates that visual training by means of a visual evoked acoustic biofeedback with Visual Pathfinder can significantly improve visual acuity and pattern reversal VEP amplitude in retinitis pigmentosa, resulting in more suitable visual performances, better quality of life, and a much more positive psychological situation for these patients.

Introduction

Retinitis pigmentosa (RP) is a leading cause of blindness and visual disability in younger people, its almost inevitable progression have always been a cause of worry for patients and a source of interest for researchers, leading to studies aimed at investigating ways of improving and/or restoring visual performance of these patients. New promising therapies for the treatment of the disease are constantly under investigation, but at present time our inability to effectively treat RP is still high, leading to an increase in the number of patients with poor visual performance who are often in a state of depression. It is for these reasons that we thought to apply biofeedback techniques to the treatment of the RP.

The biofeedback techniques used to treat patients have been around for over a quarter of a century, and the procedures themselves for over half a century. The word 'biofeedback' was coined in late 1969 to describe laboratory procedures (developed in the 1940's) that trained research subjects to alter brain activity, blood pressure, muscle tension, heart rate and other bodily functions that are not normally controlled voluntarily. At the time, many scientists looked forward to the day when biofeedback would give us a major degree of control over our bodies. They thought, for instance, that we might be able to 'will' ourselves to be more creative by changing the patterns of our brain waves. Some believed that biofeedback would one day make it possible to do away with drug treatments that often cause uncomfortable side effects in patients with high blood pressure and other serious conditions.

Although most people initially viewed these practices with skepticism, researchers proved that many individuals could alter their involuntary responses by being 'feed back' information either visually or audibly about what was occurring in their bodies.

Today, research has demonstrated that biofeedback can help in the treatment of many diseases and painful conditions. It has shown that we have more control over so-called involuntary bodily functions than we once thought possible. But it has also shown that nature imposes some limits on the extent of such control. Scientists are now trying to determine just how much voluntary control we can exert over bodily processes.

Techniques of biofeedback (BF) are used to obtain control of involuntary functions. Through these methods, adopted in various branches of medicine, the patient learns in successive stages to: (a) appreciate the variations of a bodily function through a system that measures and converts these in acoustic and/or luminous signals; (b) modify these signals and, therefore, the function connected to them; (c) automatically control the function through practice even in the absence of the return signal. [1]

There are two types of biofeedback; direct and indirect. In the former the patient can directly measure the bodily function or process to be controlled, for instance, to appreciate muscular tension through electromyographic technique connected to an appropriate device. On the other hand, indirect BF is when the patient cannot directly evaluate the bodily function but has to control this by monitoring a connected activity. An example of this is learning to sense emotional alterations through changes in perspiration.

BF techniques applied to vision are still being studied both in its methodological and physiological aspects.

Giorgi, Contestabile, Mezawa et al. and Vingolo et al. have all proposed different visual rehabilitation techniques and instruments using biofeedback strategies starting from basic systems like Accomotrack Vision Trainer (which is a high- speed infrared optometer which records the vergence of light reflected from the retina at a rate of 40 Hz, than converts the signal into an auditory tone which increases in pitch and rate as accommodation decreases; the subject listens to the tone and thus receives immediate auditory feedback as to his/ her accommodative status) or improved biofeedback integrated system (IBIS) devices, merging to more complex instruments as the fundus related MP-1 microperimeter (Nidek Technologies, Padua, Italy).

Recently introduced techniques, such as microperimetry by scanning laser ophthalmoscope (SLO), as reported by Fujii and Nilsson, and microperimtry by Mp-1 as reported by Vingolo, together with the ongoing research targeting the neurophysiology and neuro-modelling lead us to a better knowledge of the cognitive processes of rehabilitation and can serve as a useful diagnostic and therapeutic tool for the treatment of retinal disease.

Visual training with visually evoked assisted biofeedback has been used to improve performance in high speed drivers or precision shooters [7,8]. Computer programmes for visual stimulation have been used to treat amblyopia, offering to shift the apparative visual training into the domestic sphere [9,10]. Several randomized control studies on vision training systems, consisting of a background stimulation by a drifting sinusoidal grating combined with a foreground game aimed at maintaining attention have been reported in this field. Furthermore visual training has also been used to improve the saccadic performance in dyslexic children with deficitary eye movement control [11], indicating that daily practice improved not only perceptual capacity, but also voluntary saccade control, within 3 to 8 weeks. After training, the group of dyslexics was no longer statistically different from the control group.

However, at present, knowledge regarding BF applied to vision is very poor and it has never been applied to retinitis pigmentosa.

The purpose of the current study was to investigate the effect of the visual training with the acoustic biofeedback technique of the Visual Pathfinder (LACE inc.) on the evolution of retinitis pigmentosa, on the changes in visual acuity, pattern reversal visual evoked potentials and on visual performance on daily living activities of patients with retinitis pigmentosa. Our goal was to ascertain if this procedure could be useful in improving and consequently partially restoring the visual performance in these patients.

Materials and Methods

From January to April 2007 we enrolled 15 patients (8 males and 7 females, age range 8-55) with different inheritance and durations of retinitis pigmentosa (RP), and examined a total of 30 eyes, who had come to Department of Ophthalmology at the Inherited Retinal Diseases Unit of the **Policlinico Umberto I, at the "La Sapienza" University of Rome.**

Procedures were fully explained to all subjects and informed consent to participate in the study was obtained from all the patients. The ethics committee of our institution approved the study protocol. All the procedures adhered to the tenets of the Declaration of Helsinki.

The diagnosis of RP was based on a case history of slow and progressive reduction of visual acuity with nictalopia, progressive reduction of peripheral visual field documented by manual perimetry or conventional perimetry by Humphrey Field Analyzer (Humphrey 10-2 program, Goldman III stimuli, Sita Standard strategy on 68 points) typical ERG and visual evoked potential (VEP) changes, chorioretinal pigment migration, thinning of the retinal vessels, optical sub-atrophy, typical vitreal modifications.

Inclusion criteria were: patients with a visual acuity better than 0.50 logMAR with best correction, so that patient was able to maintain fixation during the examination, visual field $\geq$ **3 degree diameter circle.**

Exclusion criteria were: patients with a visual field $\leq$ **3 degree diameter** circle and/or a visual acuity worse than 0,50 logMAR with the best correction, **because of patients' inability to maintain fixation.** Direct and indirect ophthalmoscopy and three-mirror contact lens biomicroscopy were used for the exact evaluation of the macular area. Only patients who had no alterations such as cystoid macula edema or epiretinal membrane in the macular area were included in the study.

None of the patients displayed any glaucomatous or lens changes that may have affected visual acuity.

We elaborated a Visual Training Protocol which consisted of:

- 22-item questionnaire on daily living activities and patients' expectations from visual training, designed to confirm the priority task and identify any other residual functional skills requiring rehabilitation;
- assessment of distant and near best corrected visual acuity (BCVA) with a Snellen chart. All Snellen acuity scores were converted into units of log minimum angle of resolution (logMAR) values when calculating descriptive and analytical statistics;
- assessment of pattern reversal visual evoked potentials (VEP), carried out according ISCEV standard. We have chosen to assess the residual

visual capacity of RP patients by recording the pattern visual evoked potentials, because it is a useful method to provide information on the residual function of the foveal area as demonstrated by Janàky et al. Various evidence indicates that PVEPs are elicited predominantly from the central 10 degree diameter circle of the visual field [13,14], which is well preserved for a long period during the progression of RP. Projection from the central retina is received by the visual cortex overlying the occipital brain surface [15]. This part of the cortex is responsible for central vision and has a strong relationship to visual acuity. The Metrovision (France) equipment was used for stimulation and detection of the VEP responses. Black and white checkerboard **patterns with checksizes of 15' of visual angle served as the stimulus.** The viewing distance was 100 cm and the visual field extension of the stimulus display **was 17' vertically and 17' horizontally. The mean** luminosity of the stimulus pattern was set at approximately 50 cd/mq. Before the tests, the refraction was determined and corrected for viewing distance. The reversal rate was 0,5 Hz. Filters were set **between 0,5 and 80 Hz. The contrast was 70%. The patients' pupils** were undilated. Monocular stimulation was applied. The recording electrode (gold cup) was placed on the Oz site, the reference electrode on the Fz site, the ground electrode on the Fpz site. For the characterization of VEP the P100 amplitude was used. For statistical analysis the responses of each eye were analysed separately. Data are presented as means ± SD.

- 10 training sessions of 10 minutes for each eye, performed once a week using the equipment of the Visual Pathfinder (LACE inc.). Patients were asked to look at TV monitor and the consequent pattern VEP flicker guided the sound stimulation as can be seen in Figure 1. This way the patients are stimulated to maintain the highest sound (allowed by their clinical condition) and consequently the highest VEP amplitude, resulting in a training to achieve and maintain the best visual function possible. The checkerboard size used for stimulation depended on the actual visual acuity of the patient, so that the higher was the visual acuity the higher was the spatial frequency, divided in 9 levels.

- to avoid a "learning effect", the first training session was repeated twice, starting with the better eye;

- assessment of distant visual acuity and pattern reversal VEP were repeated at the end of the visual training (i.e. after 10 weeks).

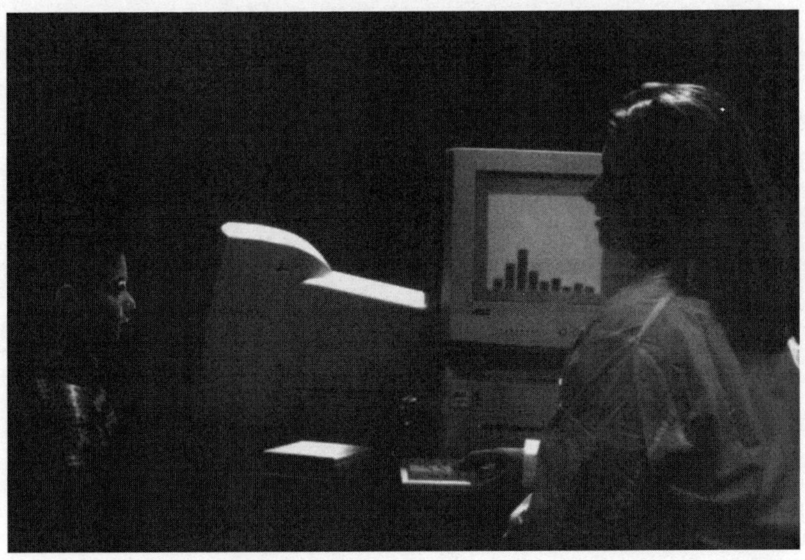

Figure 1. The picture shows the Visual Pathfinder (LACE inc.) equipment, while a child is performing his training session. Explanation in the text.

All the procedures were followed on a monitor and the results stored in a computer and on diskettes. Statistical analysis was performed using Student's t-test. P values less than 0.05 were considered statistically significant.

Results

Visual Acuity

The mean BCVA was 0.67±0.14 logMAR at the baseline assessment and 0.84±0.11 logMAR at the end of visual training; this result was statistically significant (p=0.035) as can be seen in Figure 2.

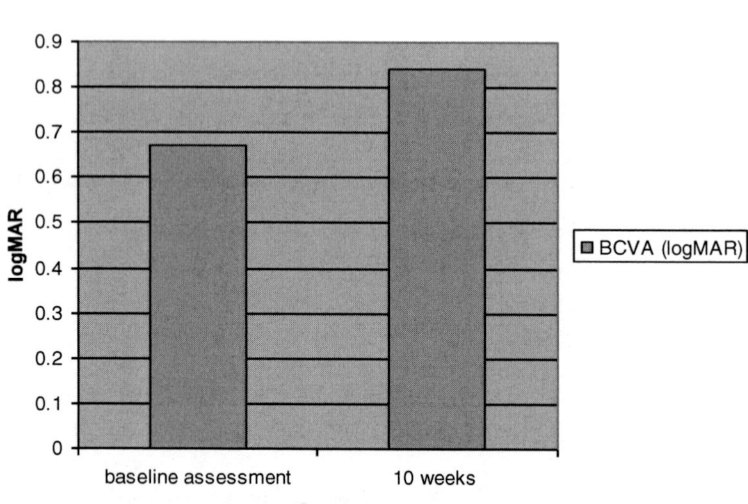

Figure 2. The picture shows the improvement in best corrected visual acuity obtained in our group of patients after 10 weeks training with the Visual Pathfinder.

Pattern Reversal Visual Evoked Potentials P100 Amplitudes

At the end of visual training, VEP P100 amplitudes improved in 10 patients, remained unchanged in 4 patients and worsened in 1 patient as can be seen in figure 3. Figure 4 shows the improvement obtained in two of the examined patients after the biofeedback training. VEP amplitudes of P100 wave was $2.14\pm0.88\mu V$ at the baseline assessment and $4.86\pm1.12\mu V$ at the end of the visual training; this result was statistically significant($p=0.012$) as can be seen in Figure 5.

To avoid the statistical disturbance due to a different VEP measurement we evaluated single cases relating actual amplitude on basal amplitude multiplied for 100, so we had a percentage showing the change in VEP amplitude.

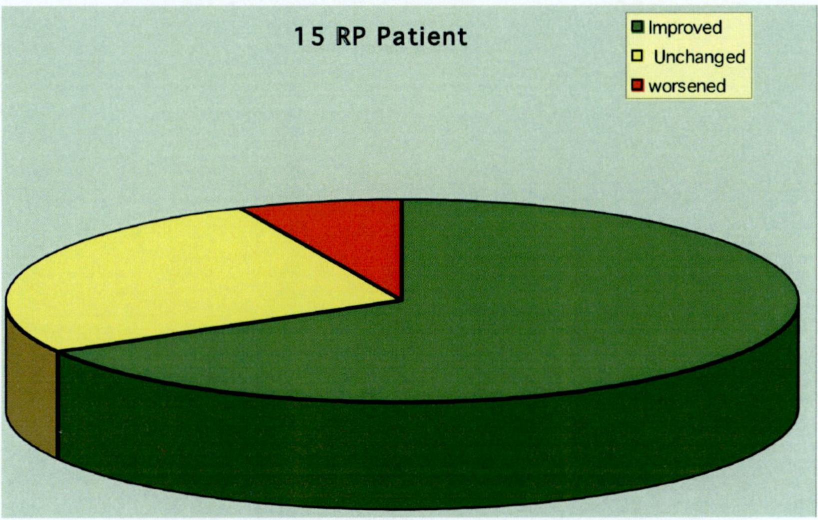

Figure 3. The pictures shows the results regarding pattern reversal visual evoked potentials P100 amplitudes. Explanation in the text.

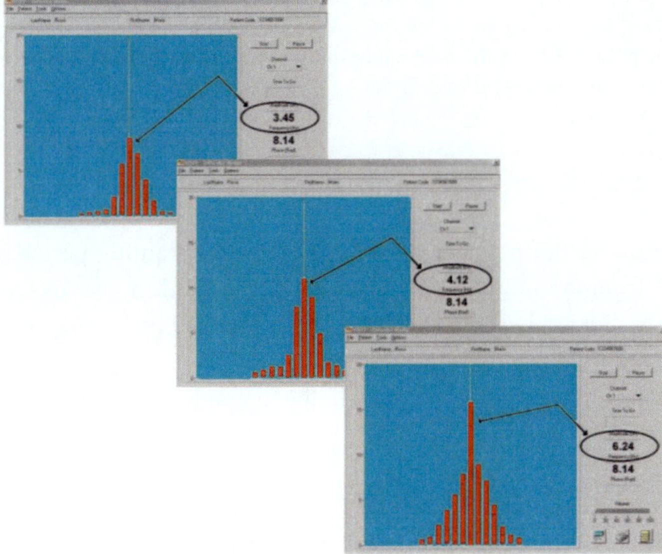

Figure 4. The pictures shows the results obtained in a patient enrolled in the study. Explanation in the text.

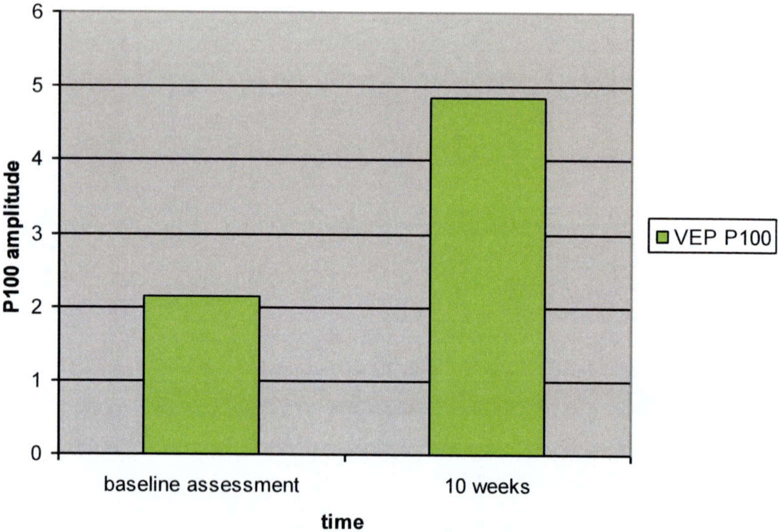

Figure 5. The picture shows the increasing in the amplitude of the P100 wave after 100 weeks training with the Visual Pathfinder.

Subjective Changes

The first question patients were asked after the training **period was: "did you benefit from the training?"**. They were then asked to give examples from everyday life concerning changes after the training. Lastly, they were asked: **"did your reading improve after training?"**

As regards subjective changes, all the patients were satisfied with the training.

Conclusion

Biofeedback is a psychophysiological way to voluntary control a non-voluntary parameter, this usually is done by an acoustic modulation of the parameter. This has been suggested in several reports on non-ophthalmologic data as demonstrated by Nakao, who suggested that biofeedback intervention may be effective in controlling mild hypertension, especially when the patient has no organ damage, explaining this result with the sympathetic activity that seems to play an important role in the differentiated response. As found by Mezawa auditory biofeedback can be useful for the treatment of congenital nystagmus patients, all the patients studied reported a subjective improvement and an improvement of foveation time, amplitude, and frequency at the end of the visual training. He theorized that this improvement could be referred to a facilitation of fixation ability due to acoustic biofeedback.

In a preliminary study Contestabile examined 18 eyes of 13 patients with low-vision who underwent visual rehabilitation with a new instrument for biofeedback (improved biofeedback integrated system (Ibis)): she demonstrated an increase in visual performances (visual acuity, colour vision, automated perimetry, contrast sensitivity and flash VEP) in contrast to a control group in which no treatment was performed. Giorgi examined 110 patients (179 eyes) with reduced visual acuity caused by different ocular disorders who underwent visual rehabilitation with improved biofeedback integrated system (Ibis) and found that visual acuity improved in 130/179 eyes (72.62%).

Several studies demonstrated that stimulation with drifting sinusoidal gratings combined with a foreground game aimed at maintaining attention improves the visual acuity of amblyopic eyes in a specific way [11,17,18]. This effect might be accounted for a synergy of spatial and temporal frequency in form versus motion channels. This method has been developed for the treatment of 'delayed' amblyopia in the elder child. It is aimed to support and complement occlusion therapy. However, the reported results obtained over 10 days should be estimated only within the context of evaluation. By no means should the results be interpreted as a renewed pledge for a short-term treatment of amblyopia.

The effects of auditory biofeedback on visual training was also used in myopia [19,20] to improve visual acuity (VA) and psychological distress evaluated in a controlled prospective study involving 55 mildly myopic (< or = -3.5 D) high school students, divided into 2 groups, matched for age and dioptric defect: 33 were treated with visual training and 22 were not, results of this study showed that VA in treated myopes improved significantly when measured by the conventional optotype, but remained unchanged when measured by computer. Psychometric scores improved significantly in the treated myopes and in the emmetropic controls.

Objectively the autorefractometer showed that 38% of the myopes had voluntary control of positive accommodation, i.e., the ability to increase spherical defect; no voluntary control of negative accommodation was observed. An increase in VA was associated with a significant increase in the foveation time (i.e., the period of time when the target is imaged on the fovea and the eye is motionless), and was partly attributable to a learning effect. The Authors concluded that biofeedback visual training had a positive effect on psychological distress and subjective VA improvement, but failed to reduce the existing myopia or delay its evolution.

Three month visual training programme was conducted in Spain [8], in which Pre-test and post-test results obtained for pistol shooting, visual function, and psychological and physical states, indicated significant gains in visual function and pistol shooting scores after the programme, while psychological (anxiety) and physical condition remained the same. Some conclusive statements can be made with regard to the relation of visual function improvement and shooting performance increment, after analysing the data. This improvement is evident in statistically significant post-test gains in the following variables: 'phoria at distance, recovery points in fusional reserves at distance, analytical amplitude, negative relative accommodation, saccadic fixations, and accommodative facility at distance and at near. The rest of the controlled visual variables also showed clinical improvement.

Although the effects of specialized training in visual analysis of skills are well documented, whether the effects are lasting or not is still unclear. Several studies on volleyball [21] or soccer players [22] showed that subjects exposed to visual training remained significantly better at diagnosing errors one year later as compared to those subjects who had not received visual training.

At present, knowledge regarding BF applied to vision is very poor and it has never been applied to pathologies such as retinitis pigmentosa.

In tapetoretinal degenerations even if the outer retina is partially destroyed inner associative systems are usually well conserved. In this view training via alternative pathways (i.e. horizontal cells or amacrine cells) could be possible, obtaining a considerable increase of visual performances for the higher amount of not regularly involved but yet stimulated pathways. The foveal projection is magnified in the cortex, which may promote the processing of information [12], another factor which might help the vision of RP patients is the dual representation of the macula in the two occipital cortices [15]. An information deficit caused by a field defect in one eye may be compensated from the other eye. Further, corresponding field defects could result in scotoma, but the brain is capable of compensating the missing part of the field ("filling- in' phenomenon) [23]. **The magnification of the foveal projection,** the double representation of the macula in the cortex and the filling- in phenomenon may account for the visual recovery by means of biofeedback techniques.

Various hypotheses regarding the mechanisms of visual function improvement after visual training techniques can be put forth. There could be improvement in ocular motor control and in 'searching capacity'. Furthermore, learning to use eccentric fixation could be a mechanism contributing to amelioration. [24] Another suggestion is an increase in the discriminating capacities both of the retina and the visual cortex and associated areas.[25] In particular it is very important to note that visual function could be improved because patients undergoing training improve their ability to demonstrate their best visual acuity and other visual abilities.

Surely a certain role in the determination of the results could be due to subjective variables such as learning effect, motivation, level of attention, psycho-physical capacities and influence of the examiner.

Andrade has shown that patients are usually unaware of their scotoma because, when the retina is damaged by a local lesion (induced scotoma), the cortical neurons driven by stimuli originating in this region do not remain inactive but become selective to stimuli originating in other parts of the retina. This process occurs in two distinct steps, each with its own time scale: i) a fast redistribution of receptive fields (RFs) in the area of the lesion and ii) a long-term reorganization that leads to the final RF configuration. Although the mechanisms underlying the slow rearrangement are becoming clearer, the first step remains obscure. Cortical neurons located in the retinotopic position corresponding to the scotoma receive some degree of activity from the unimpaired neurons in the area surrounding the lesion; Andrade and Safran demonstrated that over time these weak connections are gradually reinforced and the system eventually evolves into a new stable state, in which every neuron once again receives the same amount of activity from the source layer.

When visual acuity in the better eye worsens in patients with binocular macular diseases, they sense an improvement of vision in the fellow eye. Since each cerebral hemisphere is stimulated by both monocular and binocular neurons, this improvement can be explained by the fact that activation in areas of residual vision, which are systematically stimulated with light, increases and patients are able to perceive visual stimuli in parts of the field that had previously been unresponsive or in which superthreshold stimuli had not been detected as demonstrated by Poggel.

Another example of cerebral plasticity is blindsight, which was defined by Weiskrantz as a condition in which patients with damage in their primary visual cortex or its afferents retain the ability to detect, discriminate and locate visual stimuli presented in areas of the visual field in which they claim to be blind.

Cerebral plasticity is likely to play an important role. The audio feedback can, by increasing attentional modulation, help the brain to memorize the final fixation location. Neurons are thus able to respond to weaker stimuli than they responded to without attention. Alpeter demonstrated that attention also increases the coherence between neurons responding to the same stimulus.

Sound perception increases the conscious attention of the patient as found by Alpeter and Buia, thereby facilitating the lock-in of the visual target and increasing the permanence time of the target itself on the retina. This mechanism facilitates stimuli transmission between intraretinal neurons as well as between the retina and brain, where the highest degree of stimuli processing takes place, thus supporting a "remapping phenomenon".

Rudolph demonstrated that after brain lesions in rats the increased potentiation of subcortical inputs after cortical lesions opens a window for facilitated early functional reorganization by repetitive visual training.

In experimental studies Recovery of discrimination responding was better after auditory pulse rate training than after visual training. These data suggest that visual cortex lesions [7, 9, 33] in the rat disrupt perceptual or associational functions involving the temporal features of a visual stimulus. In addition, generalization of relational properties during cross-modal training through multimodal CNS structures appears to enhance recovery of behaviour after brain insult.

Vrensen showed a partial recovery in visual function after visual training in rats and that increase in visual ability has also been demonstrated either in adaptation-dependent conditions or after experimental photoreceptor damage, as demonstrated either in chimaeric rd mice and wild-type genotypic combination or in heterozygotic (RDS/+)mice. In these studies in surviving rod inner segment was recorded an increase in number of synaptic ribbons and presence of increased number in profiles of second order neurons processes.

The use of techniques of biofeedback in cases where conventional treatment cannot give further results presents an interesting alternative. Visual training may be considered as a rehabilitative technique towards improving residual vision.

Our experience with visual training by means of Visual Pathfinder (LACE inc.) in retinitis pigmentosa patients suggests that even if is not possible in humans, at the present time, to regenerate retinal photoreceptor, it could be possible restore in patients a better quality of sight and a positive psychologyc situation; thus even if not determines a significative change in expectance of the patient may cause a better usefulness of his performances. All treated patients showed a good response after the treatment and asked us for new sessions after a period of time.

At present it is not yet possible to advance a valid scientific theory on the true psycho-physiological mechanisms of action which make training with Visual Pathfinder and other methods of biofeedback useful. Our results undoubtedly show a rather unexpected amelioration in visual acuity and pattern reversal VEP.

Improvement through BF training in patients who are afflicted with pathologies which remain either stable or worsen, where traditional treatment cannot offer further results, is of interest and well worthy of attention. Further study in this field is warranted.

References

[1]   Contestabile, MT; Recupero, SM; Palladino, D; De Stefanis, M; Abdolrahimzadeh, S; Suppressa, F; Balacco Gabrieli, C. A new method of biofeedback in the management of low vision. *Eye.*, 2002, 16(4), 472-80.

[2]   Giorgi, D; Contestabile, MT; Pacella E, Gabrieli, CB. An instrument for biofeedback applied to vision. *Appl. Psychophysiol Biofeedback.*, 2005, 30(4), 389-95.

[3]   Mezawa, M; Ishikawa, S; Ukai, K. Changes in waveform of congenital nystagmus associated with biofeedback treatment. *Br. J. Ophthalmol.*, 1990, 74(8), 472-6.

[4]   Vingolo, EM; Cavarretta, S; Domanico, D; Parisi, F; Malagola, R. Microperimetric biofeedback in AMD patients. *Appl. Psychophysiol Biofeedback.*, 2007, 32(3-4), 185-9.

[5]   Fujii, GY ; De Juan E, Jr ; Sunness, J ; Humayun, MS ; Pieramici, DJ ; Chang, TS; Patient selection for macular translocation surgery using the scanning laser ophthalmoscope. *Ophthalmology.*, 2002, 109, 1737-44.

[6]   Nilsson, UL ; Frennesson, C ; Nilsson, SE. Patients with AMD and a large absolute central scotoma can be trained successfully to use eccentric viewing, as demonstrated in a scanning laser ophthalmoscope. *Vision Res.*, 2003, 43(16), 1777-87.

[7]   Wood, JM; Abernethy, B. An assessment of the efficacy of sports vision training programs. *Optom. Vis. Sci.*, 1997, 74(8), 646-59.

[8]   Quevedo i Junyent L, Sole i Forto J. Visual training programme applied to precision shooting. *Ophthalmic Physiol. Opt.*, 1995, 15(5), 519-23.

[9]   Delay, ER. Cross-modal transfer effects on visual discrimination depends on lesion location in the rat visual system. *Physiol. Behav.*, 2001, 73(4), 609-20.

[10]   Luo, J; Zhang, X; Zhang, LN. Study of visual training of amblyopia *Zhonghua Hu Li Za Zhi.*, 1996, 31(3), 144-5.

[11]   Fischer, B; Hartnegg, K. Effects of visual training on saccade control in dyslexia. *Perception.*, 2000, 29(5), 531-42.

[12]   Janàky, M; Pàlffy, A; Horvàth, G; Tuboly, G; Benedek, G. Pattern-reversal electroretinograms and visual evoked potentials in retinitis pigmentosa. *Doc. Ophthalmol.*, 2008, 117(1), 27-36.

[13]   Sakaue, H; Katsumi, O; Mehta, M; Hirose, T. Simultaneous pattern reversal ERG and VER recordings. Effect of stimulus field and central scotoma. *Invest. Ophthalmol. Vis. Sci.*, 1990, 31, 506–511.

[14]   Regan, D. Evoked potentials in psychology, sensory physiology and clinical medicine. 1972. Chapman and Hall, London.

[15]   Horton, JC; Hoyt, WF. The representation of the visual field in human striate cortex. A revision of the classic Holmes map. *Arch. Ophthalmol.*, 1991, 109, 816–824.

[16]   Nakao, M; Nomura, S; Shimosawa, T; Fujita, T; Kuboki, T. Blood pressure biofeedback treatment, organ damage and sympathetic activity in mild hypertension. *Psychother. Psychosom.*, 1999, 68(6), 341-7.

[17]   Kampf, U; Muchamedjarow, F; Seiler, T. Supportive amblyopia treatment by means of computer games with background stimulation, a placebo controlled pilot study of 10 days *Klin. Monatsbl. Augenheilkd.*, 2001, 218(4), 243-50.

[18]   Marsh, E; Baker, R. Normal and adapted visuooculomotor reflexes in goldfish. J. *Neurophysiol.*, 1997, 77(3), 1099-118.

[19]   Rupolo, G; Angi, M; Sabbadin, E; Caucci, S; Pilotto, E; Racano, E; de, Bertolini, C. Treating myopia with acoustic biofeedback, a prospective

study on the evolution of visual acuity and psychological distress. *Psychosom Med.*, 1997, 59(3), 313-7.

[20] Angi, MR; Caucci, S; Pilotto, E; Racano, E; Rupolo, G; Sabbadin, E. Changes in myopia, visual acuity, and psychological distress after biofeedback visual training. *Optom. Vis. Sci.*, 1996, 73(1), 35-42.

[21] Wilkinson, S. Effects of training in visual discrimination after one year, visual analysis of volleyball skills. *Percept. Mot. Skills.*, 1992, 75(1), 19-24.

[22] Hitzeman, SA; Beckerman, SA. What the literature says about sports vision. *Optom. Clin.*, 1993, 3(1), 145-69.

[23] Ramachandran, VS; Gregory, RL. Perceptual filling in of artificially induced scotomas in human vision. *Nature.*, 1991, 350, 699–702.

[24] Trachtman, JN. Raccolta dei Risultati Ottenuti in Pazienti a Seguito del Trattamento con l'Allenatore Della Vista Accomotrack Vision Trainer-Riduzione Della Miopia Atti del XVI corso di aggiornamento Apimo. *Montecatini Terme.*, Italy, 1994, 183-195.

[25] D'Andrea, P. Risultati della Rieducazione Visiva in un Caso di Maculopatia, *Valutazioni Campimetriche Atti SIRV*, Roma, Italy, 1995, 37-46.

[26] Andrade, MA; Muro, EM; Moran, F. Simulation of plasticity in the adult visual cortex. *Biol. Cybern.*, 2001, 84, 445-51.

[27] Safran, AB; Landis, T. Plasticity in the adult visual cortex, implications for the diagnosis of visual field defects and visual rehabilitation. *Curr. Opin. Ophthalmol.*, 1996, 7, 53-64.

[28] Poggel, DA; Kasten, E; Sabel, BA. Attentional cueing improves vision restoration therapy in patients with visual field defects. *Neurology* 2004, 63, 2069-2076.

[29] Kentridge, RW; Heywood, CA; Weiskrantz, L. Spatial attention speeds discrimination without awareness in blindsight. *Neuropsychologia* 2004, 42, 831-835.

[30] Alpeter, E; Mackben, M; Trauzettel-Klosinski, S. The importance of sustained attention for patients with maculopthies. *Vision Research* 2000, 40, 1539-1547.

[31] Buia, C; Tiesinga, P. Attentional modulation of firing rate and synchrony in a model cortical network. *J. Comput. Neurosci.*, 2006, 20, 247-64.

[32] Rudolph, TM; Delay, ER. Recovery of a temporally based visual discrimination after visual cortex lesion in the rat. *Behav. Brain Res.*, 1993 Feb 26, 53, 189-99.

[33] Vrensen, G; Cardozo, JN. Changes in size and shape of synaptic connections after visual training, an ultrastructural approach of synaptic plasticity. *Brain Res.*, 1981, 218, 79-97.

Index

B

D

E

F

M

macrophages, 115, 171, 188

macular degeneration, 3, 49, 123, 125, 134, 147, 182

maintaining attention, 194, 201

maintenance, 20, 21, 54, 129, 169

males, 76, 194

malondialdehyde, 166

mammals, 42

management, 105, 136, 205

manners, 78

manufacturer, 95, 152

marriage, 96

marrow, x, 2, 3, 11, 15, 24, 27, 28, 55, 56, 57, 79, 86, 120, 125

mask, 171

matrix, xiv, 51, 114, 116, 140, 141, 143, 144, 150, 154, 156, 157, 160, 169, 174, 179, 180, 181, 182, 183, 184, 185, 186, 187, 188, 189, 190

matrix metalloproteinase, xiv, 140, 141, 179, 180, 181, 183, 184, 185, 187, 188, 189, 190

maturation, x, 2, 10, 11, 13, 14, 59

measurement, 19, 198

measures, 193

media, 34

mediated gene delivery, 21

mediators, 145, 181

medicine, 183, 193, 206

melanoma, 189

membranes, xv, 115, 141, 142, 146, 150, 159, 168, 176, 177, 183

memory, 75

mesenchymal stem cells, 55, 59

mesenchymal stromal cells, 51

messenger RNA, 78

metabolic, 67, 77, 79, 108, 128, 136, 186

metabolism, 119

metabolites, 151

metal ions, 144

metalloproteinase, xiv, 140, 141, 179, 180, 181, 183, 186, 187, 188, 189, 190

metalloproteinases, 179, 181, 182, 183, 184, 185, 187, 188

metazoans, 77

methionine, 121

mice, 28, 50, 51, 57, 60, 78, 79, 91, 107, 108, 121, 122, 123, 146, 147, 148, 149, 152, 153, 169, 175, 179, 183, 189, 204

microarray, 104, 105, 109, 119

microarray technology, 105

microenvironment, 28

microglia, xiii, 112, 115, 120, 123, 125, 147, 159, 187, 189

microglial cells, 123, 147, 182

microRNAs (miRNAs), 77

microscope, 6

microsurgery, 92

microtubule, 18, 68, 77

migration, xi, xiii, 25, 65, 66, 112, 114, 115, 117, 120, 123, 145, 171, 187, 190, 195

mirror, 195

misfolding, xi, 65, 68

mitochondria, 145, 150, 168, 176, 177

mitochondrial, 146, 150, 151, 173, 176, 178, 185

mitochondrial membrane, 178

mitosis, 50

mitotic, 48, 118

MMP-2, xiv, 140, 144, 145, 146, 149, 151, 154, 156, 157, 160, 161, 163, 165, 167, 169, 171, 172, 179

MMP-3, 146

MMP-9, xiv, 140, 143, 145, 149, 150, 151, 154, 156, 157, 160, 161, 163, 165, 167, 169, 171, 172, 173, 174, 177, 179, 180, 181, 184, 187, 190

MMPs, xiv, xv, 140, 141, 143, 145, 149, 150, 151, 159, 167, 168, 169, 171, 173, 174, 175, 176, 177, 187, 188

modalities, 116

models, xiii, 49, 51, 77, 79, 84, 85, 87, 91, 112, 118, 119, 120, 124, 128, 183

O

P

Q

R

S

T

.wustl.edu/course/eyeret.html,   B.   S